Head and Neck Cancer Clinics

Series editors
Rehan Kazi
Head and Neck Cancer
Manipal University
Manipal, India

Raghav C. Dwivedi
Head and Neck Cancer
Royal Marsden Hospital
London, United Kingdom

Head and Neck Cancer (HNC) is a major challenge to public health. Its management involves a multidisciplinary team approach, which varies depending on the subtle differences in the location of the tumour, stage and biology of disease and availability of resources. In the wake of rapidly evolving diagnostic technologies and management techniques, and advances in basic sciences related to HNC, it is important for both clinicians and basic scientists to be up-to-date in their knowledge of new diagnostic and management protocols. This series aims to cover the entire range of HNC-related issues through independent volumes on specific topics. Each volume focuses on a single topic relevant to the current practice of HNC, and contains comprehensive chapters written by experts in the field. The reviews in each volume provide vast information on key clinical advances and novel approaches to enable a better understanding of relevant aspects of HNC. Individual volumes present different perspectives and have the potential to serve as stand-alone reference guides. We believe these volumes will prove useful to the practice of head and neck surgery and oncology, and medical students, residents, clinicians and general practitioners seeking to develop their knowledge of HNC will benefit from them.

More information about this series at http://www.springer.com/series/13779

K. Alok Pathak • Richard W. Nason
Editors

Controversies in Oral Cancer

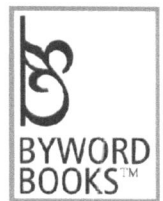

BYWORD
BOOKS™

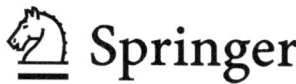
Springer

Editors
K. Alok Pathak
Head and Neck Surgical Oncology
Cancer Care Manitoba
Winnipeg
Canada

Richard W. Nason
Surgery
University of Manitoba
Winnipeg
Canada

ISSN 2364-4060   ISSN 2364-4079   (electronic)
Head and Neck Cancer Clinics
ISBN 978-81-322-3448-7   ISBN 978-81-322-2574-4   (eBook)
DOI 10.1007/978-81-322-2574-4

Springer New Delhi Heidelberg New York Dordrecht London

Cover illustration by Dan Gibbons DCR(R), PgCert(CT)

Printed on acid-free paper

Springer (India) Pvt. Ltd. is part of Science+Business Media (www.springer.com)

This series is dedicated to the research and charity efforts of Cancer Aid and Research Foundation (CARF), Mumbai, India (www.cancerarfoundation.org).

Foreword and a Note on the Series

Oral cancer is one of the most common forms of head and neck cancer and not surprisingly still has several debatable grey areas and controversies. This volume of HNCC series on *Controversies in Oral Cancer* is timely and addresses some of the key issues in the management of oral cancer. This volume has been compiled by internationally renowned experts Drs. Pathak and Nason, who have contributed immensely to the field. The chapters on novel molecular targets, potentially malignant diseases of the oral cavity, management of N0 neck, mandible-preserving alternatives, current options in reconstruction of the oral cavity, and surveillance after treatment of oral cancers are particularly interesting.

Head and neck cancer (HNC) is a major public health challenge. Its management involves a multidisciplinary team approach, which varies depending upon the subtle differences in the location of the tumour, stage and biology of disease, and availability of resources. In the wake of rapidly evolving diagnostic technologies and management techniques, and advances in the basic sciences related to HNC, it is important for both clinicians and basic scientists to be up-to-date in their knowledge of new diagnostic and management protocols.

This series aims to cover the entire range of HNC-related issues through independent volumes on specific topics. Each volume focuses on a single topic relevant to the current practice of HNC and contains comprehensive chapters written by experts in the field. The reviews in each volume provide vast information on key clinical advances and novel approaches to enable a better understanding of relevant aspects in HNC.

Individual volumes present different perspectives and have the potential to serve as stand-alone reference guides. We believe these volumes will prove useful for the practice of head and neck surgery and oncology. Medical students, residents, clinicians and general practitioners seeking to develop their knowledge of HNC will benefit from them.

London, UK   Raghav C. Dwivedi
Manipal, India   Rehan Kazi

Preface

Oral cancer is the sixth most common cancer worldwide and causes a significant burden on society. As is evident throughout this monograph, considerable progress is being made in the understanding of this disease and its treatment. Understanding the molecular basis for this cancer has contributed to new treatment strategies using novel molecular targets. The signs of early changes in the oral mucosa that may herald the onset of oral cancer are now more completely understood, leading to early detection and timely intervention. There have been considerable advances in the traditional treatment modalities of surgery, radiation, and chemotherapy and their use in combination. In spite of these advances, oral cancer still presents at a relatively advanced stage, the increments in overall survival have been small, and the considerable morbidity that accompanies treatment adversely affects the quality of life. Controversy in this area is therefore inevitable and was important in stimulating development of this volume of Head and Neck Cancer Clinics.

This volume brings together the work of experts from clinical and basic sciences specialties and addresses some of the controversial issues and advances in the management of oral cancer. Improving the outcome for the oral cancer patient will require dedicated work from many disciplines working together as multidisciplinary units.

Winnipeg, Canada	K. Alok Pathak
Winnipeg, Canada	Richard W. Nason

Abbreviations

3–D	3-Dimensional
5–FU	5-Fluorouracil
AC	Adenocarcinoma
ALT	Anterolateral thigh flap
ASHNS	American Society for Head and Neck Surgery
ATP	Adenosine triphosphate
BERA	Brainstem-evoked response audiometry
Carbo	Carboplatin
Cetux	Cetuximab
CIVI	Continuous intravenous infusion
COPD	Chronic obstructive pulmonary disease
COX-2	Cyclooxygenase-2
CRT	Chemo-radiotherapy
CSC	Cancer stem cell
CSF	Cerebrospinal fluid
CT	Chemotherapy
CTA	CT angiography
CT scan	Computerized tomography scan
CUP	Carcinoma of unknown primary
EAC	External auditory canal
EEA	Expanded endonasal approach
EGFR	Epidermal growth factor receptor
EGFRvIII	EGFR variant III
EORTC	European Organization for Research and Treatment of Cancer
EXTREME	Erbitux in First-Line Treatment of Recurrent or Metastatic Head and Neck Cancer (trial)
FDA	Food and Drug Administration
FGF	Fibroblast growth factor
GPCR	G protein-coupled receptor
H&E	Haematoxylin and eosin
HCV	Hepatitis C virus
HDAC	Histone deacetylase
HNC	Head and neck cancer

HNSCC	Head and neck squamous cell carcinoma
HPV	Human papillomavirus
IFN-α	Interferon alpha
IgA	Immunoglobulin A
IGF-1R	Insulin-like growth factor-1 receptor
IMF	Infrahyoid myocutaneous flap
IMRT	Intensity-modulated radiation therapy
IP	Inverted papilloma
mAb	Monoclonal antibody
MALT	Mucosa-associated lymphoid tissue
MRA	Magnetic resonance angiography
MRI	Magnetic resonance imaging
mTOR	Mammalian target of rapamycin
NCCN	National Comprehensive Cancer Network
NFκB	Nuclear factor kappa B
OLP	Oral lichen planus
OS	Overall survival
Pac	Paclitaxel
PacPF	Paclitaxel, cisplatin + 5-fluorouracil
PDGF	Platelet-derived growth factor
PDGFR	Platelet-derived growth factor receptor
PEG	Percutaneous endoscopic gastrostomy
PET	Positron emission tomography
PF	Cisplatin + 5-fluorouracil
PKB	Protein kinase B
PMD	Potentially malignant disorder
PMMF	Pectoralis major myocutaneous flap
PTEN	Phosphatase and tensin homologue
Q-time	Quality-adjusted survival time
QoL	Quality of life
RET	REarranged during Transfection
RFF	Radial forearm flap
RMT	Retromolar trigone
RT	Radiotherapy
RTK	Receptor tyrosine kinase
RTOG	Radiation Therapy Oncology Group
SBT	Skull base tumour
SCC	Squamous cell carcinoma
SHNS	Society of Head and Neck Surgery
SS	Sjögren syndrome
STAT	Signal transducer and activator of transcription
STIR	Short tau inversion recovery
SWOG	Southwest Oncology Group
TENS	Transcutaneous electric nerve stimulation
TFG-α	Transforming (tumour) growth factor-alpha

TFG-β	Transforming (tumour) growth factor-beta
TK	Tyrosine kinase
TPF	Taxotere (docetaxel), cisplatin + 5-FU
TSH	Thyroid stimulating hormone
TTF	Time to treatment failure
VAS	Visual analogue scale
VEGF	Vascular endothelial growth factor
VEGFR	Vascular endothelial growth factor receptor
VP	Ventriculo-peritoneal
XI	Xerostomia inventory

Contents

1 Potential Molecular Targets: From Bench to Bedside   1
Ajay Matta and Ranju Ralhan

2 Potentially Malignant Disorders of the Oral Cavity 17
David C. Williams and William T. McGaw

3 Mandible-Preserving Alternatives 33
K. Alok Pathak, Rehan Kazi, and Richard W. Nason

4 Surgical Management of Oral Cancer 45
Richard W. Nason and K. Alok Pathak

5 Management of the N0 Neck in Oral Cancer 51
Richard W. Nason and K. Alok Pathak

**6 Current Options and Controversies in Reconstruction
of the Oral Cavity** 61
Ravi Sachidananda and S. Mark Taylor

7 Challenges in Preserving Salivary Gland Functions 79
Rashmi Koul and Arbind Dubey

**8 Systemic Therapies in the Management of Head
and Neck Cancer** 99
Andrew W. Maksymiuk

9 Surveillance After Treatment of Oral Cancer 115
Richard W. Nason and K. Alok Pathak

Index 121

Contributors

Arbind Dubey Department of Radiation Oncology, University of Saskatchewan, Staff Radiation Oncologist, Allan Blair Cancer Centre, Regina, SK, Canada

Rehan Kazi Head and Neck Cancer, Manipal University, Manipal, India

Rashmi Koul Department of Radiation Oncology, University of Saskatchewan, Staff Radiation Oncologist, Allan Blair Cancer Centre, Regina, SK, Canada

Andrew W. Maksymiuk Medical Oncology, CancerCare Manitoba, Department of Internal Medicine, University of Manitoba, Winnipeg, MB, Canada

Ajay Matta Department of Chemistry and Centre for Research in Mass Spectrometry, York University, Toronto, ON, Canada

William T. McGaw Division of Oral Medicine and Pathology, University of Alberta, Edmonton, AB, Canada

Richard W. Nason Department of Surgery, Faculty of Medicine, University of Manitoba, Winnipeg, MB, Canada

K. Alok Pathak Head and Neck Surgical Oncology, CancerCare Manitoba, Department of Surgery, University of Manitoba, Winnipeg, MB, Canada

Ranju Ralhan Department of Otolaryngology – Head and Neck Surgery, University of Toronto and Joseph and Mildred Sonshine Family Centre for Head and Neck Diseases, Mount Sinai Hospital, Toronto, ON, Canada

Ravi Sachidananda Head & Neck Surgery and Microvascular Reconstruction, QE2 HSC, VG Site, Halifax, NS, Canada

S. Mark Taylor Otolaryngology, Head & Neck Surgery, Facial Plastic and Reconstructive surgery, QE2 HSC, VG Site, Halifax, NS, Canada

David C. Williams Division of General Surgery, 2D4.39 Walter Mackenzie Health Sciences Center, Edmonton, AB, Canada

Potential Molecular Targets: From Bench to Bedside

Ajay Matta and Ranju Ralhan

Introduction

HNSCC is the sixth most common cancer, accounting for ~600,000 new cases and more than 300,000 deaths annually worldwide [1]. The non- surgical management of HNSCC has undergone major changes, including technological advances in radiation delivery for reducing normal tissue toxicity and increasing the dose to tumour tissue [2–6], as well as demonstrating the superiority of concomitant chemoradiotherapy (CRT) over RT alone in definitive [7] and adjuvant settings [8, 9]. Improvements in CRT, such as the establishment of concurrent platinum-based CT with external beam RT as the gold standard of primary treatment, as well as the addition of induction CT and altered fractionation regimens, have increased both survival rates and organ preservation [10, 11]. Moreover, advances in imaging have allowed for the development of techniques, such as intensity-modulated RT, which deliver high doses of radiation precisely to tumours while sparing surrounding tissue [12]. Despite these improvements in treatment strategies, the prognosis of HNSCC patients in advanced stages (III/IV) remains largely unsatisfactory owing to locoregional recurrence and dose-limiting toxicities, or to the increased risk of cardiac failure in cancer patients, which limits the clinical utility of these strategies [13, 14].

A. Matta
Department of Chemistry and Centre for Research in Mass Spectrometry,
York University, 4700 Keele Street, Toronto, ON M3J 1P3, Canada

R. Ralhan (✉)
Department of Otolaryngology – Head and Neck Surgery,
University of Toronto and Joseph and Mildred Sonshine Family Centre for Head and Neck Diseases, Mount Sinai Hospital,
Joseph and Wolf Lebovic Health Complex, 600 University Avenue, Room 6-500,
Toronto, ON M5G 1X5, Canada
e-mail: rralhan@mtsinai.on.ca

© The Author(s) 2012
K.A. Pathak, R.W. Nason (eds.), *Controversies in Oral Cancer*,
Head and Neck Cancer Clinics, DOI 10.1007/978-81-322-2574-4_1

Several epigenetic and genetic events, viz. aberrant expression and/or function of regulators of the cell cycle, growth and signalling, apoptosis, motility, angiogenesis and microRNAs are implicated in the pathogenesis of HNSCCs and constitute plausible targets for therapy. Advances in epigenomics, genomics, proteomics, bioinformatics and integration of all this knowledge have provided a holistic understanding of signalling pathways and networks that regulate cellular functions, intra- and intercellular communication, and tumour-host interactions. Deregulation of signalling pathways (including EGFR, Ras, nuclear factor kappa B [NFκB], STAT3, Wnt/β-catenin, TGF-β, and PI3-K/Akt/mTOR) contribute to the development of HNSCC [15, 16]. Among these proteins, the potential drug targets currently being studied in clinical trials include EGFR, VEGF, serine/threonine kinases and associated proteins (E6 and E7) of human papillomavirus (HPV). This chapter discusses the efficacy and limitations of inhibitors targeting these proteins and how the emerging information on cross-talks between different signalling pathways can help to understand the limited efficacy of mono-targeted therapies for HNSCC. In turn, this knowledge can be harnessed for developing novel, multiple molecular-targeted strategies for HNSCC treatment.

Molecular-Targeted Therapies for HNSCC

HNSCC cells have the ability to exploit diverse signalling pathways for growth advantage, cell survival and evasion of apoptosis. Figure 1.1 shows a schematic representation of the signalling pathways deregulated in HNSCC and the agents targeting key components. Several molecular pathways have been targeted in HNSCC for the development of novel therapies. Different aetiological factors and risk habits can result in distinct genetic and epigenetic alterations, which may trigger different signalling pathways that impact development and progression of HNSCCs. A proof of principle is the constitutive activation of Ras/Raf/MAPK pathway caused by Ras mutations in the areca quid-chewing oral cancers, whereas in cancers associated with chronic tobacco exposure, this pathway is likely to be activated downstream from EGFR activation [17, 18]. Another evidence of multiple aberrant pathways is the altered NFκB function leading to activation of STAT3 by an autocrine or paracrine mechanism initiated by interleukin (IL)-6 release, independent from EGFR [19, 20]. In addition, *de novo*/acquired chemo-resistance is a significant problem in the management of HNSCCs. The emerging data suggest that cancer stem cells (CSCs) may be responsible for acquired resistance to CT/RT in HNSCCs. CSCs are a subpopulation of cells that can self-renew and produce differentiated cells that form the bulk of the tumour [21–23]. It is proposed that the current HNSCC treatment regimens selectively kill the differentiated cancer cells producing tumour regression, but do not eliminate the CSCs. Understanding the molecular signatures of HNSCC stem cells will define new targets for designing novel therapeutic strategies. These targeted therapies offer new treatment strategies even for heavily pre-treated and terminally ill cancer patients who become unresponsive or are unable to tolerate CT or RT.

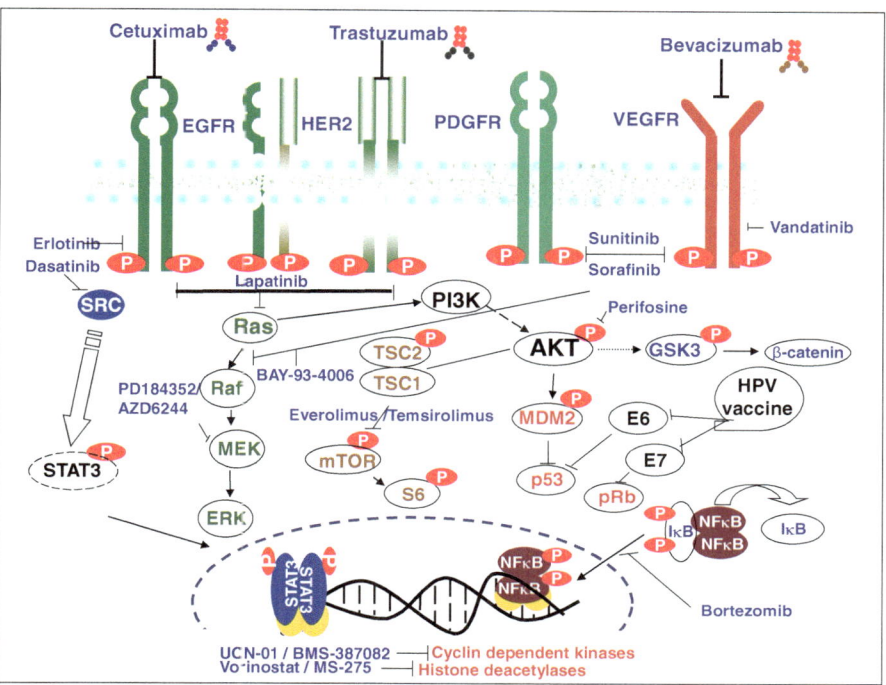

Fig. 1.1 Signalling pathways frequently deregulated in HNSCC, the molecular targets involved and their corresponding inhibitors as potential anticancer agents. EGFR and VEGFR signals utilize a variety of downstream molecular pathways including the PI3-K-Akt-mTOR, STAT and Ras-MAPK (*ERK*) pathways. Agents targeting these pathways include the monoclonal antibodies cetuximab, panitumumab and bevacizumab; tyrosine kinase inhibitors including erlotinib, vandetanib and lapatinib; multikinase inhibitors such as sorafenib and sunitinib; Src family kinase inhibitors dasatinib and saracatinib; mTOR inhibitors such as everolimus and temsirolimus; and nucleic acid decoy, namely, STAT3 decoy. *EGFR* epidermal growth factor receptor, *VEGFR* vascular endothelial cell growth factor receptor

EGFR and VEGFR signals utilize a variety of downstream molecular pathways, including the PI3-K-Akt-mTOR, STAT and Ras-MAPK (ERK) pathways. The clinical efficacies of the inhibitors targeting important pathways regulated by EGFR, VEGF and Akt have been reviewed [24–31]. Agents targeting these pathways include the following (Table 1.1): (i) Monoclonal antibodies (mAbs), namely cetuximab, panitumumab, necitumumab, ch806 and bevacizumab; (ii) tyrosine kinase (TK) inhibitors, including erlotinib, gefitinib, vandetanib and lapatinib; (iii) multikinase inhibitors, such as sorafenib and sunitinib; (iv) Src family kinase inhibitors, such as dasatinib and saracatinib; (v) mTOR inhibitors, such as everolimus and temsirolimus; and (vi) STAT3 decoy. Large amounts of preclinical *in vitro* and *in vivo* data have been obtained on the anti-proliferative properties of these inhibitors, both as single agents and in combination with CT/RT. The inclusion of these agents in combined modality treatment regimens for early and/or advanced stage HNSCC

Table 1.1 Molecular targets and their inhibitors used for HNSCC therapy

Molecular target/ inhibitor	Type	Mechanism of action	Dose-limiting toxicities
(I) Erb family (EGFR, HER2, HER3 and HER4)			
Cetuximab	Recombinant human/mouse chimeric IgG1 monoclonal antibody	Binds EGFR and inhibits activation of receptor tyrosine kinase (RTK) Stimulates receptor internalization and down-regulation from the cell surface	Acne-like rashes, fever and chills, asthaenia, transaminase level increase, nausea
Pertuzumab	Humanized mAb for HER2	Inhibits ligand-activated HER dimerization with HER2, thus inhibiting activation of intracellular signalling	Acne-like rashes
Panitumumab	Humanized EGFR mAb (IgG2)	Binds to extracellular domains of EGFR	Acne formation
Martuzumab	Humanized EGFR mAb (IgG1)	Binds to extracellular domains of EGFR	Headache and fever
Trastuzumab	HER2/neu antibody	Complement- and antibody-dependent cell-mediated cytotoxicity	Cardiac dysfunction, renal failure, membranous nephropathy and glomerulonephritis
(II) Tyrosine kinase			
Gefitinib	Synthetic small molecule	Targets EGFR tyrosine kinase domain	Skin rash, diarrhoea, nausea and emesis
Erlotinib	Synthetic small molecule	Inhibitor of EGFR	Skin rashes, dry skin and diarrhoea
Lapatinib	Synthetic small molecule	Inhibits EGFR and HER2/neu heterodimer	Diarrhoea, nausea, fatigue and anorexia
(III) VEGF			
Bevacizumab	Humanized recombinant mAb	Antibody directed against VEGF	Hypertension, proteinuria, bleeding and thrombosis
(IV) Multikinase inhibitor			
Sorafenib	Synthetic molecule	Serine/threonine Raf-1 kinase; receptor tyrosine kinases, including EGFR, PDGFR, KIT and Flt3	Hypothyroidism
BIBF 1120	Synthetic molecule	Inhibitor of VEGF, PDGF and FGF	Nausea, vomiting, diarrhoea, abdominal pain, fatigue and asymptomatic, reversible liver enzyme elevations
Sunitinib	Synthetic molecule	Inhibits PDGFR, EGFR, stem cell factor receptor (KIT) and Flt, HER2/neu	–

(continued)

Table 1.1 (continued)

Molecular target/ inhibitor	Type	Mechanism of action	Dose-limiting toxicities
Vandetanib (ZD6474)	Synthetic molecule	Inhibitor of VEGFR, EGFR, and rearranged during transfection (RET) tyrosine kinases	–
(V) PI3K/Akt/mTOR			
Temsirolimus	Synthetic molecule	mTOR	–
(VI) HSP90 inhibitor			
Geldanamycin	Benzoquinone ansamycin antibiotic	Degrades HSP90	–
(VII) Proteasome inhibitor			
Bortezomib	Synthetic molecule	Proteasome inhibitor	Peripheral neuropathy, neutropenia and thrombocytopenia

FGF fibroblast growth factor, *PGDF* platelet-derived growth factor, *PGDFR* platelet-derived growth factor receptor

is likely to increase therapeutic efficacy. Consequently, several targeted agents are under clinical trials in HNSCC, with many phases I/II studies already completed and some phase III studies in progress (reviewed in Refs. [24–33]).

Epithelial growth factor receptor (EGFR) overexpression is observed in more than 90 % of HNSCCs and its activation has been reported to influence the resistance to RT and/or CT in HNSCCs, making it the most plausible therapeutic target [34–39]. Two primary strategies under investigation as EGFR-targeted therapies include: (i) Inhibition of the extracellular ligand binding using humanized mAbs, and (ii) inhibition of its TK domain with a small molecule. The binding of epithelial growth factor (EGF) or transforming growth factor alpha (TGFα) to its receptor (EGFR) results in the formation of homodimers or heterodimers with other members of the Erb family (Her2/neu, Erb3, Erb4) which activates the downstream signalling cascades-Ras/Raf/MAPK and the PI3-K/Akt/mTOR pathways (Fig. 1.1). The activation of these signalling events is responsible for tumorigenesis by regulating proliferation and inhibition of apoptosis, growth and survival, and cell adhesion/motility. Thus, competing EGF or TGFα for binding to its receptor, using mAbs as antagonists, is considered as the most appropriate approach for inhibition of EGFR signalling. However, mAbs designed against the extracellular domain of EGFR, such as cetuximab, pertuzumab, panitumumab and trastuzumab, have shown limited efficacy in monotherapy. Cetuximab was approved by the Food and Drug Administration (FDA) in 2006 as the first molecular-targeted therapy for HNSCC on the basis of a phase III trial that demonstrated significant improvements in locoregional control and survival with this mAb compared with RT alone [40].

A recent update from this study demonstrated that cetuximab plus RT provided a sustained survival benefit of ~9 %, and compared favourably with the 6.5 % benefit shown by platinum-based CT plus RT [41, 42]. The combination of cetuximab with 5-fluorouracil (5-FU) and carboplatin/cisplatin showed increased survival with no cumulative toxicity in a phase I/II trial in recurrent HNSCC [43–45]. Cetuximab has been shown to act as a tumour-specific radiosensitizer in recurrent or metastatic disease, although it has also been demonstrated to be effective in second-line treatment of metastatic and recurrent HNSCC patients as monotherapy [46–50]. The toxic effects of cetuximab are less severe than those observed with conventional CT, RT or both; the addition of cetuximab to any of these regimens has no effect on compliance, as shown in the Erbitux in First-Line Treatment of Recurrent or Metastatic Head and Neck Cancer (EXTREME) trial [43]. The quality-of-life assessment of patients from the EXTREME trial demonstrated that addition of cetuximab to 5-FU and a platinum compound significantly improved patients' overall quality of life without any adverse effect on social functioning [43]. Thus, the replacement of cisplatin with cetuximab or future biological agents as the standard of care for HNSCC patients is increasingly being considered [51]. Importantly, only a subset of HNSCC patients respond to EGFR targeting, despite the increased expression of EGFR; no correlation has been reported between EGFR overexpression and clinically meaningful response to EGFR inhibitors [31, 37, 52]. Constitutive activation of the Ras/Raf/MAPK, STAT3 and PI3-K/Akt/mTOR signalling pathways independent of EGFR by other stimuli [such as hypoxia, Ras activation or phosphatase and tensin homologue (PTEN) mutation and inhibition] has been reported recently and might account for the failure of clinical response to EGFR inhibitors [52, 53]. The presence of constitutively activated EGFR variant III (EGFRvIII) in HNSCCs may also account for resistance to EGFR inhibition by mAbs [54]. Acquired resistance to cetuximab is accompanied by EGFR internalization/degradation and subsequent EGFR-dependent activation of Her3 [55]. Thus, the best combination of methods for use of EGFR as a drug target remains to be determined. Panitumumab is a fully humanized antibody that is likely to overcome the dose-dependent toxicity of cetuximab. However, this antibody is less immunogenic than cetuximab and may reduce the production of neutralizing antibodies against the drug, as well as reduce the incidence of life-threatening hypersensitivity reactions [56, 57]. Currently, two phase III trials of panitumumab are under way. Moreover, clinical trials of trastuzumab reported increased chances of cardiomyopathy in HNSCC patients undergoing treatment [58]. Zalutumumab (fully humanized IgG1 mAb) and nimotuzumab (humanized murine IgG1 mAb) are under phase III trials in HNSCC patients [59].

The other EGFR-targeted therapies, including EGFR-targeted TK inhibitors, have yet to demonstrate efficacy in a phase III study. TK inhibitors (such as gefitinib, erlotinib and lapatinib) block the adenosine triphosphate (ATP) pocket of EGFR, thereby inhibiting phosphorylation and downstream signal transduction. However, gefitinib has not shown marked success in clinical trials for HNSCC [60–65]. Erlotinib is in active development for HNSCC, demonstrating encouraging results in several studies [66–69]. A multicentric study showed that erlotinib was well tolerated in pre-treated HNSCCs and prolonged disease-free survival [66]. Lapatinib has dual specificity for EGFR and Her-2, and is currently under evaluation as an adjuvant to postoperative CRT in a phase III trial. An important mechanism that has been explained to overcome EGFR inhibition by erlotinib/gefitinib is epithelial–mesenchymal transition [70, 71]. In addition, cross-talks between EGFR and cell adhesion molecules, cytokine receptors, ion channels and G protein-coupled receptor (GPCR) lead to the activation of EGFR [72, 73]. Together these mechanisms explain why most clinical trials suggest no correlation between EGFR protein expression and response to EGFR inhibitors. Tumour signalling pathway components that work synergistically with EGFR or compensate for the loss of EGFR-initiated signalling are likely to be ideal targets for multi-targeted therapy. Erb family-targeted and Src family-targeted agents are in clinical development [74]. Thus, drug candidates targeting cellular pathways other than EGFR are under active development following a model based on the design of EGFR-targeted therapies. The main aims of clinical studies investigating non-EGFR-based therapies include: (i) Establishing efficacy as an adjuvant to CRT or cetuximab; (ii) determining toxicities; and (iii) recording data on factors influencing prognosis and response to therapy.

PI3-K/Akt Pathway as a Molecular Target for Therapy

Uncontrolled activation of the PI3-K/Akt/mTOR pathway contributes to the development and progression of HNSCC and is an important target to counteract resistance to RT and/or CT [75]. PTEN deletions and 'hot-spot' mutations of the PI3-K gene have been shown to possess transforming capacity *in vitro* and *in vivo*; hence restoration of mutated or absent PTEN activity might be a target for Akt inhibition. Protease inhibitors downregulate the phosphorylation and expression of active PI3-K, which is responsible for radioresistance in HNSCC. Activation of Akt has been proposed as the mechanism of resistance to EGFR inhibitors. Therefore, combining Akt inhibitors with anti-EGFR agents may be useful in effective management of HNSCC. The mammalian target of rapamycin (mTOR) regulates cell growth, proliferation, motility, survival, protein synthesis and transcription. Rapamycin derivatives (such as everolimus, temserolimus and deforolimus) are potent inhibitors of mTOR and do not share the problems of poor solubility and chemical stability of rapamycin. A clinical trial using cisplatin and everolimus (RAD-001) in HNSCC is in progress [76]. However, not all HNSCCs have an activated PI3-K/Akt/mTOR pathway; hence, molecular signatures need to be developed to define patients who may benefit from inhibitors of this pathway. Moreover, mTOR inhibition blocks the natural negative feedback on insulin-like growth factor-1 receptor (IGF-1R) signalling impinging on PI3-K. This results in increased PI3-K and Akt activation which could potentially counteract the inhibition of mTOR. Dual inhibition of both IGF-1R signalling or TK inhibitors and mTOR may result in a superior antiproliferative effect over each single strategy in HNSCCs [77, 78]. However, the major limitation of mTOR inhibitors in clinical trials is their dose-limiting toxicity. Hence, when combined with mTOR inhibitors, natural products (e.g. curcumin) that hit multiple cellular targets, including mTOR, may reduce the toxic side-effects and augment clinical efficacy.

Vascular endothelial growth factor receptor (VEGFR): Increased expression of VEGF and its receptors in HNSCCs underscores their importance in angiogenesis and survival of tumour cells under hypoxic conditions [79, 80]. VEGF expression is regulated by hypoxia-inducible factor-1 alpha-dependent and -independent processes, both of which involve PI3-K and Akt. Targeting of angiogenesis by inhibition of the VEGF ligand itself and small molecule inhibition of VEGFR TKs are two strategies being investigated for molecular-targeted therapy of HNSCC [81–83]. Bevacizumab, a humanized VEGF mAb, binds and sequesters all five isoforms of VEGF and not only inhibits angiogenesis, but also facilitates the increased delivery of chemotherapeutic agents by decreasing microvascular permeability and decreasing intra-tumour pressure [83]. The single-agent anti-angiogenic drugs have not shown promising activity in unselected HNSCC patients, with a response rate of <4 %. On the other hand, combinations of bevacizumab with erlotinib showed a response rate of 14.6 %. Studies of bevacizumab with CT (phase III Eastern Cooperative Oncology Group trial) and in combination with CRT are currently in progress [84, 85]. However, HNSCCs show inter-tumoral angiogenic heterogeneity; in-depth understanding of the variability of angiogenic phenotype within a given HNSCC is important for designing cytokine-targeted anti-angiogenic therapies. Another potential strategy is inhibition of VEGFR by small molecule inhibitors of TK inhibitors. Vandetanib, sunitinib and sorafenib are the three VEGFR-targeted TK inhibitors under investigation for HNSCC with discordant results, which emphasizes that criteria for selecting patients will be critical for limiting toxicity in future studies [86–88].

Kinases (Serine/Threonine and Tyrosine) as Potential Molecular Targets

Sorafenib, an oral multikinase inhibitor, targets serine/threonine Raf-1 kinase and receptor TKs (RTKs)—VEGFR, platelet-derived growth factor (PDGF) receptor, KIT and Flt3. Phase II trials in patients with recurrent or metastatic HNSCC showed that sorafenib was well tolerated with modest anticancer activity, comparable to monotherapy [86–89]. BIBF 1120 targets VEGF, PDGF, fibroblast growth factor (FGF) receptor and Src family of TKs (Src, LcK, Lyn). Vandetanib (ZD6474), an inhibitor of VEGFR, EGFR, and rearranged during transfection (RET) TKs, is being tested in HNSCC as monotherapy and also in combination with RT [88]. Dasatinib (BMS-354825) and sarcatinib (AZD0530), which are synthetic, small molecule inhibitors of Src family kinases that are currently in clinical evaluation for HNSCC, also inhibit protein TKs—bcr-abl, EphA2, and PDGFβ [89]. However, a major challenge in the development of multikinase inhibitors is the rapid evolution of mutant inhibitor-resistant kinases. Therefore, appropriate multitargeted inhibitors or combinations need to be planned in advance of clinical application.

Other Biological-Targeted Agents for HNSCC

Biological agents, pemetrexed and enzastaurin (an oral protein kinase C beta inhibitor) in combination with cisplatin are showing considerable promise and no unexpected toxicities in phase I trials [90, 91]. Aurora kinase A inhibitor and paclitaxel in combination are also under investigation for HNSCC management [92]. Among the new cyclooxygenase-2 (COX-2) inhibitors, salvianolic acid B has shown promise for HNSCC prevention and treatment [93]. Geldanamycin analogues have demonstrated potent inhibition of Hsp90, demonstrating significant anti-tumour activity in both cell culture and animal studies. Bortezomib inhibits activation of NFκB and sensitizes these cells to chemotherapy, radiation, or immunotherapy without added toxicities [94–97]. Histone deacetylases (HDACs) are enzymes that regulate the acetylation of histone and non-histone proteins, including p53, p21 and NFκB. Altered expressions of HDACs have been reported in several human malignancies, including HNC. Inhibitors of HDAC, such as suberoylanilide hydroxamic acid, have been shown to induce growth arrest, differentiation and promote apoptosis of HNSCC cell lines [98]. HDAC inhibitors target NFκB and also increase radiosensitivity, and thus may be tried in future trials. STAT3 is a member of a family of transcription factors which regulates the expression of several critical cellular processes, viz. cell growth, migration and inhibition of apoptosis, and acts as a downstream target from EGFR [99–101]. The clinical development of small molecule inhibitors of STAT3 has been challenging; a proof of concept for a soluble nucleic acid decoy for the STAT3 promoter in HNSCC is currently being investigated in a phase 0 study.

Human Papillomavirus Vaccines

Little attention has been paid to understanding the effect of HPV on therapeutic response to targeted agents in HNSCC. It is increasingly being recognized that the molecular pathogenesis of HPV-infected oropharyngeal SCC exhibits marked geographical variation and is different from tobacco- and alcohol-associated HNSCC [102, 103]; so how can these biologically different tumours show the same response to targeted agents? In fact, HPV-associated HNSCC shows better prognosis than HPV-negative tumours, although the molecular basis of improved prognosis is not clearly understood. In future trials, evaluation of HPV status of HNSCC patients is likely to provide better insight into the outcome of clinical response to targeted agents. In addition, HPV-positive tumours may possess additional molecular therapeutic targets, such as the E6 and E7 proteins that would be used for designing novel strategies for the management of HPV-positive HNSCC.

Future Strategies

The complexity of the aberrant signalling in HNSCC as shown in Fig. 1.1 explains why interfering with only single steps in these pathways has not shown marked clinical response in HNSCC patients. The development of new biological agents should focus on inhibitors that are likely to hit multiple targets. Alternatively, a combination of different agents that target distinct specific pathways is likely to inhibit the escape of tumour cells by alternate mechanisms, leading to more effective disease control. The success of future clinical trials will depend upon the selection of the patient population and a study design for assessing response to therapy. Further, to evaluate the efficacy of these biological agents, there is an urgent need to identify novel biomarkers that can be used to accurately assess and individualize therapy. In addition, the elucidation of mechanisms of resistance to targeted therapies is also likely to improve outcomes by identifying new potential drug and diagnostic targets as well as lead to a rational combination of multi-targeted therapies. Patients having advanced locoregional disease or recurrent/metastatic HNSCC have been often selected for conducting phase II clinical trials. Most of these patients develop multifactorial resistance, having received RT/CT/CRT for treatment of primary tumours, and therefore are less likely to respond to new agents effectively. Thus, testing of new agents as first-line therapy is likely to show better clinical response than if used as second-line therapy in recurrent/metastatic HNSCC patients. Moreover, cumulative resistance observed in recurrent/metastatic HNSCC patients limits the generalization of clinical response to patients with early disease for target validation.

The feasibility of conducting translational research is often hampered by the ethical constraints in obtaining tumour biopsies. Evaluation of new compounds in a preoperative window setting will bring a paradigm shift in the design of phase II trials. Biopsies collected at the time of diagnosis, and before or after treatment, or at the time of surgery, or before locoregional therapy will enable evaluation of predictive molecular markers and may help in identifying subgroups of patients most likely to respond to therapy (or develop primary resistance). Furthermore, these paired tumour specimens will also provide insights into the pharmacodynamics of novel agents, and help understand their mechanism of action. Adequate documentation of the specificities of inhibitors and observed toxicities in a database in phase I and phase II studies would constitute a valuable resource for identifying cellular targets whose inhibition should be avoided. Assessment of clinical response dependent on progression-based end-points will provide a more realistic evaluation of the efficacy of biological agents. Specific molecular markers may give a more objective evaluation of clinical response. To cite an example, pharmacodynamic tissue studies conducted in a phase I/II trial of erlotinib and cisplatin in patients with recurrent or metastatic HNSCC showed that high EGFR gene copy in tumour specimens may predict which patients are likely to respond to erlotinib, and decreased p-EGFR level in skin biopsies during therapy may represent a potential surrogate marker for improved clinical outcome. Multidimensional scaling represents a novel way to evaluate these relationships between molecular markers and clinical outcome. This may be used for the evaluation of clinical efficacy of anti-angiogenic agents by measuring intra-tumoral blood flow perfusion parameters using molecular imaging or dynamic control-enhanced CT/magnetic resonance imaging (MRI).

More predictive tumour models and better ways to monitor target inhibition in humans in a minimally invasive manner are needed. As cell culture and animal models are severely limited in mimicking the development of human HNSCC, there is an urgent need to develop minimally invasive methods to discover and monitor biomarkers for evaluation of HNSCC in humans. New imaging modalities in conjunction with proteomic technologies may be investigated to monitor changes in signalling proteins and metabolites. Early detection technologies may allow us to diagnose and exterminate tumours before their acquisition of survival capabilities that empower them with resistance to therapy.

In conclusion, molecular-targeted therapies are promising novel treatment options for HNSCC patients. EGFR-targeted therapies have shown significant but limited efficacy. Inhibitors of angiogenesis, proteasomes and multifunctional TKs are under evaluation as single agents, or in combination with CT/RT or CRT. Several questions regarding dosing, combination and patient selection remain to be addressed. Nonetheless, molecular-targeted therapies will complement CT/RT or CRT in HNSCC patients in future. An in-depth understanding of how the complex cellular signalling cascades and networks are reprogrammed in HNSCC and in the presence of mono-targeting inhibitors is vital to rational designing of combinations of inhibitors. Innovative trial designs and appropriate patient selection are critical for the success of new trials to translate molecular-targeted therapies from the bench to the clinic. Coordination between the development of molecular-targeted therapies and biomarkers for assessment of their clinical efficacy can achieve the promise of personalized medicine for HNSCC patients.

Competing Interests The authors declare that they have no competing interests.

References

1. Jemal A, Siegel R, Xu J, *et al.* Cancer statistics, 2010. *CA: A Cancer Journal for Clinicians* 2010;**60**:277–300.
2. Lee NY, Le QT. New developments in radiation therapy for head and neck cancer: Intensity-modulated radiation therapy and hypoxia targeting. *Semin Oncol* 2008;**35**:236–50.
3. Guerrero Urbano T, Clark CH, Hansen VN, *et al.* A phase I study of dose-escalated chemoradiation with accelerated intensity modulated radiotherapy in locally advanced head and neck cancer. *Radiother Oncol* 2007;**85**:36–41.
4. Bhide S, Clark C, Harrington K, *et al.* Intensity modulated radiotherapy improves target coverage and parotid gland sparing when delivering total mucosal irradiation in patients with squamous cell carcinoma of head and neck of unknown primary site. *Med Dosim* 2007;**32**:188–95.

5. Miles EA, Clark CH, Urbano MT, *et al*. The impact of introducing intensity modulated radiotherapy into routine clinical practice. *Radiother Oncol* 2005;**77**:241–6.
6. Pignon JP, Bourhis J, Domenge C, *et al*. Chemotherapy added to loco-regional treatment for head and neck squamous cell carcinoma: Three meta-analyses of updated individual data. MACH-NC Collaborative Group. Meta-analysis of chemotherapy on head and neck cancer. *Lancet* 2000;**355**:949–55.
7. Bernier J, Domenge C, Ozsahin M, *et al*. Postoperative irradiation with or without concomitant chemotherapy for locally advanced head and neck cancer. *N Engl J Med* 2004;**350**:1945–52.
8. Cooper JS, Pajak TF, Forastiere AA, *et al*. Postoperative concurrent radiotherapy and chemotherapy for high-risk squamous cell carcinoma of the head and neck. *N Engl J Med* 2004;**350**:1937–44.
9. Argiris A, Karamouzis MV, Raben D, *et al*. Head and neck cancer. *Lancet* 2008;**371**:1695–709.
10. Pignon JP, le Maitre A, Maillard E, *et al*. Meta-analysis of chemotherapy in head and neck cancer (MACH-NC): An update on 93 randomised trials and 17,346 patients. *Radiother Oncol* 2009;**92**:4–14.
11. Dirix P, Nuyts S. Evidence-based organ-sparing radiotherapy in head and neck cancer. *Lancet Oncol* 2010;**11**:85–91.
12. Budach W, Hehr T, Budach V, *et al*. A meta-analysis of hyperfractionated and accelerated radiotherapy and combined chemotherapy and radiotherapy regimens in unresected locally advanced squamous cell carcinoma of the head and neck. *BMC Cancer* 2006;**6**:28.
13. Gibson MK, Li Y, Murphy B, *et al*. Eastern Cooperative Oncology Group, Randomized phase III evaluation of cisplatin plus fluorouracil versus cisplatin plus paclitaxel in advanced head and neck cancer (E1395): An intergroup trial of the Eastern Cooperative Oncology Group. *J Clin Oncol* 2005;**23**:3562–7.
14. de Castro G Jr, Snitcovsky IM, Gebrim EM, *et al*. High-dose cisplatin concurrent to conventionally delivered radiotherapy is associated with unacceptable toxicity in unresectable, non-metastatic stage IV head and neck squamous cell carcinoma. *Eur Arch Otorhinolaryngol* 2007;**264**:1475–82.
15. Singh B. Molecular pathogenesis of head and neck cancers. *J Surg Oncol* 2008;**97**:634–9.
16. Molinolo AA, Amornphimoltham P, Squarize CH, *et al*. Dysregulated molecular networks in head and neck carcinogenesis. *Oral Oncol* 2009;**45**:324–34.
17. Warnakulasuriya KA, Ralhan R. Clinical, pathological, cellular and molecular lesions caused by oral smokeless tobacco—a review. *J Oral Pathol Med* 2007;**36**:63–77.
18. Arredondo J, Chernyavsky AI, Jolkovsky DL, *et al*. Receptor-mediated tobacco toxicity: Cooperation of the Ras/Raf-1/MEK1/ERK and JAK-2/STAT-3 pathways downstream of alpha7 nicotinic receptor in oral keratinocytes. *FASEB J* 2006;**20**:2093–101.
19. Neiva KG, Zhang Z, Miyazawa M, *et al*. Cross talk initiated by endothelial cells enhances migration and inhibits anoikis of squamous cell carcinoma cells through STAT3/Akt/ERK signaling. *Neoplasia* 2009;**11**:583–93.
20. Chen CC, Chen WC, Lu CH, *et al*. Significance of interleukin-6 signaling in the resistance of pharyngeal cancer to irradiation and the epidermal growth factor receptor inhibitor. *Int J Radiat Oncol Biol Phys* 2010;**76**:1214–24.
21. Prince ME, Ailles LE. Cancer stem cells in head and neck squamous cell cancer. *J Clin Oncol* 2008;**26**:2871–5.
22. Song J, Chang I, Chen Z, *et al*. Characterization of side populations in HNSCC: Highly invasive, chemoresistant and abnormal Wnt signaling. *PLoS One* 2010;**5**:e11456.
23. Shakib K, Schrattenholz A, Soskic V. Stem cells in head and neck squamous cell carcinoma. *Br J Oral Maxillofac Surg* 2010 Sep 8. [Epub ahead of print].
24. Sano D, Fooshee DR, Zhao M, *et al*. Targeted molecular therapy of head and neck squamous cell carcinoma with the tyrosine kinase inhibitor vandetanib in a mouse model. *Head Neck* 13 Jul 2010. [Epub ahead of print].

25. Goerner M, Seiwert TY, Sudhoff H. Molecular targeted therapies in head and neck cancer—an update of recent developments. *Head Neck Oncol* 2010;**2**:8.
26. Razak AR, Siu LL, Le Tourneau C. Molecular targeted therapies in all histologies of head and neck cancers: An update. *Curr Opin Oncol* 2010;**22**:212–20.
27. Bozec A, Peyrade F, Fischel JL, *et al.* Emerging molecular targeted therapies in the treatment of head and neck cancer. *Expert Opin Emerg Drugs* 2009;**14**:299–310.
28. Dietz A, Boehm A, Mozet C, *et al.* Current aspects of targeted therapy in head and neck tumors. *Eur Arch Otorhinolaryngol* 2008;**265**:3–12.
29. Shirai K, O'Brien PE. Molecular targets in squamous cell carcinoma of the head and neck. *Curr Treat Options Oncol* 2007;**8**:239–51.
30. Langer CJ. Targeted therapy in head and neck cancer: State-of-the-art 2007 and review of clinical applications. *Cancer* 2008;**112**:2635–45.
31. Fung C, Grandis JR. Emerging drugs to treat squamous cell carcinomas of the head and neck. *Expert Opin Emerg Drugs* 2010;**15**:355–73.
32. Cassell A, Grandis JR. Investigational EGFR-targeted therapy in head and neck squamous cell carcinoma. *Expert Opin Investig Drugs* 2010;**19**:709–22.
33. Harrington KJ, Kazi R, Bhide SA, *et al.* Novel therapeutic approaches to squamous cell carcinoma of the head and neck using biologically targeted agents. *Indian J Cancer* 2010;**47**:248–59.
34. Choong NW, Cohen EE. Epidermal growth factor receptor directed therapy in head and neck cancer. *Crit Rev Oncol Hematol* 2006;**57**:25–43.
35. Harari PM, Huang S. Radiation combined with EGFR signal inhibitors: Head and neck cancer focus. *Semin Radiat Oncol* 2006;**16**:38–44.
36. Moon C, Chae YK, Lee J. Targeting epidermal growth factor receptor in head and neck cancer: Lessons learned from cetuximab. *Exp Biol Med (Maywood)* 2010;**235**:907–20.
37. Ang KK, Andratschke NH, Milas L. Epidermal growth factor receptor and response of head-and-neck carcinoma to therapy. *Int J Radiat Oncol Biol Phys* 2004;**58**:959–65.
38. Rodemann HP, Dittmann K, Toulany M. Radiation-induced EGFR-signaling and control of DNA-damage repair. *Int J Radiat Biol* 2007;**83**:781–91.
39. Kim S, Grandis JR, Rinaldo A, *et al.* Emerging perspectives in epidermal growth factor receptor targeting in head and neck cancer. *Head Neck* 2008;**30**:667–74.
40. Bonner JA, Harari PM, Giralt J, *et al.* Radiotherapy plus cetuximab for squamous cell carcinoma of the head and neck. *N Engl J Med* 2006;**354**:567–78.
41. Bonner JA, Harari PM, Giralt J, *et al.* Radiotherapy plus cetuximab for locoregionally advanced head and neck cancer: 5-year survival data from a phase 3 randomised trial, and relation between cetuximab-induced rash and survival. *Lancet Oncol* 2010;**11**:21–8.
42. Teoh DC, Rodger S, Say J, *et al.* Hypofractionated radiotherapy plus cetuximab in locally advanced head and neck cancer. *Clin Oncol (R Coll Radiol)* 2008;**20**:717.
43. Vermorken JB, Mesia R, Rivera F, *et al.* Platinum-based chemotherapy plus cetuximab in head and neck cancer. *N Engl J Med* 2008;**359**:1116–27.
44. Pfister DG, Su YB, Kraus DH, *et al.* Concurrent cetuximab, cisplatin, and concomitant boost radiotherapy for locoregionally advanced, squamous cell head and neck cancer: A pilot phase II study of a new combined-modality paradigm. *J Clin Oncol* 2006;**24**:72–8.
45. Herbst RS, Arquette M, Shin DM, *et al.* Phase II multicenter study of the epidermal growth factor receptor antibody cetuximab and cisplatin for recurrent and refractory squamous cell carcinoma of the head and neck. *J Clin Oncol* 2005;**23**:5578–87.
46. Bourhis J, Rivera F, Mesia R, *et al.* Phase I/II study of cetuximab in combination with cisplatin or carboplatin and fluorouracil in patients with recurrent or metastatic squamous cell carcinoma of the head and neck. *J Clin Oncol* 2006;**24**:2866–72.
47. Bernier J. Drug Insight: Cetuximab in the treatment of recurrent and metastatic squamous cell carcinoma of the head and neck. *Nat Clin Pract Oncol* 2008;**5**:705–13.

48. Burtness B, Goldwasser MA, Flood W, *et al.* Phase III randomized trial of cisplatin plus placebo compared with cisplatin plus cetuximab in metastatic/recurrent head and neck cancer: An Eastern Cooperative Oncology Group study. *J Clin Oncol* 2005;**23**:8646–54.
49. Baselga J, Trigo JM, Bourhis J, *et al.* Phase II multicenter study of the antiepidermal growth factor receptor monoclonal antibody cetuximab in combination with platinum-based chemotherapy in patients with platinum-refractory metastatic and/or recurrent squamous cell carcinoma of the head and neck. *J Clin Oncol* 2005;**23**:5568–77.
50. Mesia R, Rivera F, Kawecki A, *et al.* Quality of life of patients receiving platinum-based chemotherapy plus cetuximab first line for recurrent and/or metastatic squamous cell carcinoma of the head and neck. *Ann Oncol* 2010. [Epub ahead of print].
51. Rowan K. Should cetuximab replace cisplatin in head and neck cancer? *J Natl Cancer Inst* 2010;**102**:74–6, 8.
52. Rogers SJ, Harrington KJ, Rhys-Evans P, *et al.* Biological significance of c-erbB family oncogenes in head and neck cancer. *Cancer Metastasis Rev* 2005;**24**:47–69.
53. Morgillo F, Bareschino MA, Bianco R, *et al.* Primary and acquired resistance to anti-EGFR targeted drugs in cancer therapy. *Differentiation* 2007;**75**:788–99.
54. Sok JC, Coppelli FM, Thomas SM, *et al.* Mutant epidermal growth factor receptor (EGFRvIII) contributes to head and neck cancer growth and resistance to EGFR targeting. *Clin Cancer Res* 2006;**12**:5064–73.
55. Erjala K, Sundvall M, Junttila TT, *et al.* Signaling via ErbB2 and ErbB3 associates with resistance and epidermal growth factor receptor (EGFR) amplification with sensitivity to EGFR inhibitor gefitinib in head and neck squamous cell carcinoma cells. *Clin Cancer Res* 2006;**12**:4103–11.
56. Saltz L, Easley C, Kirkpatrick P. Panitumumab. *Nat Rev Drug Discov* 2006;**5**:987–8.
57. Kim R. Cetuximab and panitumumab: Are they interchangeable? *Lancet Oncol* 2009;**10**:1140–1.
58. Guglin M, Cutro R, Mishkin JD. Trastuzumab-induced cardiomyopathy. *J Card Fail* 2008;**14**:437–44.
59. Rivera F, Vega-Villegas ME, Lopez-Brea MF, *et al.* Current situation of Panitumumab, Matuzumab, Nimotuzumab and Zalutumumab. *Acta Oncol* 2008;**47**:9–19.
60. Stewart JS, Cohen EE, Licitra L, *et al.* Phase III study of gefitinib compared with intravenous methotrexate for recurrent squamous cell carcinoma of the head and neck [corrected]. *J Clin Oncol* 2009;**27**:1864–71.
61. Cohen EE, Kane MA, List MA, *et al.* Phase II trial of gefitinib 250 mg daily in patients with recurrent and/or metastatic squamous cell carcinoma of the head and neck. *Clin Cancer Res* 2005;**11**:8418–24.
62. Caponigro F, Romano C, Milano A, *et al.* A phase I/II trial of gefitinib and radiotherapy in patients with locally advanced inoperable squamous cell carcinoma of the head and neck. *Anticancer Drugs* 2008;**19**:739–44.
63. Chua DT, Wei WI, Wong MP, *et al.* Phase II study of gefitinib for the treatment of recurrent and metastatic nasopharyngeal carcinoma. *Head Neck* 2008;**30**:863–7.
64. Hainsworth JD, Spigel DR, Burris HA III, *et al.* Neoadjuvant chemotherapy/gefitinib followed by concurrent chemotherapy/radiation therapy/gefitinib for patients with locally advanced squamous carcinoma of the head and neck. *Cancer* 2009;**115**:2138–46.
65. Argiris A, Ghebremichael M, Gilbert J, *et al.* A phase III randomized, placebo-controlled trial of docetaxel (D) with or without gefitinib (G) in recurrent or metastatic (R/M) squamous cell carcinoma of the head and neck (SCCHN): A trial of the Eastern Cooperative Oncology Group (ECOG). *J Clin Oncol* 2009;**27**(Suppl):5 s (abstract 6011).
66. Soulieres D, Senzer NN, Vokes EE, *et al.* Multicenter phase II study of erlotinib, an oral epidermal growth factor receptor tyrosine kinase inhibitor, in patients with recurrent or metastatic squamous cell cancer of the head and neck. *J Clin Oncol* 2004;**22**:77–85.
67. Siu LL, Soulieres D, Chen EX, *et al.* Phase I/II trial of erlotinib and cisplatin in patients with recurrent or metastatic squamous cell carcinoma of the head and neck: A Princess Margaret

Hospital phase II consortium and National Cancer Institute of Canada Clinical Trials Group Study. *J Clin Oncol* 2007;**25**:2178–83.

68. Kim ES, Kies MS, Glisson BS, *et al.* Final results of a phase II study of erlotinib, docetaxel and cisplatin in patients with recurrent/metastatic head and neck cancer. 2007 ASCO Annual Meeting Proceedings Part I. *J Clin Oncol* 2007;**25** (18S)(June 20 Supplement):6013.

69. Cohen EE, Rosen F, Stadler WM, *et al.* Phase II trial of ZD1839 in recurrent or metastatic squamous cell carcinoma of the head and neck. *J Clin Oncol* 2003;**21**:1980–7.

70. Frederick BA, Helfrich BA, Coldren CD, *et al.* Epithelial to mesenchymal transition predicts gefitinib resistance in cell lines of head and neck squamous cell carcinoma and non-small cell lung carcinoma. *Mol Cancer Ther* 2007;**6**:1683–91.

71. Haddad Y, Choi W, McConkey DJ. Delta-crystallin enhancer binding factor 1 controls the epithelial to mesenchymal transition phenotype and resistance to the epidermal growth factor receptor inhibitor erlotinib in human head and neck squamous cell carcinoma lines. *Clin Cancer Res* 2009;**15**:532–42.

72. Zandi R, Larsen AB, Andersen P, *et al.* Mechanisms for oncogenic activation of the epidermal growth factor receptor. *Cell Signal* 2007;**19**:2013–23.

73. Schwentner I, Witsch-Baumgartner M, Sprinzl GM, *et al.* Identification of the rare EGFR mutation p.G796S as somatic and germline mutation in white patients with squamous cell carcinoma of the head and neck. *Head Neck* 2008;**30**:1040–4.

74. Egloff AM, Grandis JR. Targeting epidermal growth factor receptor and SRC pathways in head and neck cancer. *Semin Oncol* 2008;**35**:286–97.

75. Bussink J, van der Kogel AJ, Kaanders JH. Activation of the PI3-K/AKT pathway and implications for radioresistance mechanisms in head and neck cancer. *Lancet Oncol* 2008;**9**:288–96.

76. Nathan CO, Amirghahari N, Rong X, *et al.* Mammalian target of rapamycin inhibitors as possible adjuvant therapy for microscopic residual disease in head and neck squamous cell cancer. *Cancer Res* 2007;**67**:2160–8.

77. Oh SH, Kim WY, Kim JH, *et al.* Identification of insulin-like growth factor binding protein-3 as a farnesyl transferase inhibitor SCH66336-induced negative regulator of angiogenesis in head and neck squamous cell carcinoma. *Clin Cancer Res* 2006;**12**:653–61.

78. Jimeno A, Kulesza P, Wheelhouse J, *et al.* Dual EGFR and mTOR targeting in squamous cell carcinoma models, and development of early markers of efficacy. *Br J Cancer* 2007;**96**:952–9.

79. Shang ZJ, Li ZB, Li JR. VEGF is up-regulated by hypoxic stimulation and related to tumour angiogenesis and severity of disease in oral squamous cell carcinoma: *In vitro* and *in vivo* studies. *Int J Oral Maxillofac Surg* 2006;**35**:533–8.

80. Liang X, Yang D, Hu J, *et al.* Hypoxia inducible factor-alpha expression correlates with vascular endothelial growth factor-C expression and lymphangiogenesis/angiogenesis in oral squamous cell carcinoma. *Anticancer Res* 2008;**28**:1659–66.

81. Van Meter ME, Kim ES. Bevacizumab: Current updates in treatment. *Curr Opin Oncol* 2010 Sep 1. [Epub ahead of print].

82. Seiwert TY, Cohen EE. Targeting angiogenesis in head and neck cancer. *Semin Oncol* 2008;**35**:274–85.

83. Ferrara N. Vascular endothelial growth factor as a target for anticancer therapy. *Oncologist* 2004;**9** (Suppl 1):2–10.

84. Cohen EE, Davis DW, Karrison TG, *et al.* Erlotinib and bevacizumab in patients with recurrent or metastatic squamous cell carcinoma of the head and neck: A phase I/II study. *Lancet Oncol* 2009;**10**:247–57

85. Fujita K, Sano D, Kimura M, *et al.* Anti-tumor effects of bevacizumab in combination with paclitaxel on head and neck squamous cell carcinoma. *Oncol Rep* 2007;**18**:47–51.

86. Elser C, Siu LL, Winquist E, *et al.* Phase II trial of sorafenib in patients with recurrent or metastatic squamous cell carcinoma of the head and neck or nasopharyngeal carcinoma. *J Clin Oncol* 2007;**25**:3766–73.

87. Sano D, Kawakami M, Fujita K, *et al.* Anti-tumor effects of ZD6474 on head and neck squamous cell carcinoma. *Oncol Rep* 2007;**17**:289–95.
88. Gustafson DL, Frederick B, Merz AL, *et al.* Dose scheduling of the dual VEGFR and EGFR tyrosine kinase inhibitor vandetanib (ZD6474, Zactima) in combination with radiotherapy in EGFR-positive and EGFR-null human head and neck tumor xenografts. *Cancer Chemother Pharmacol* 2008;**61**:179–88.
89. Johnson FM, Saigal B, Talpaz M, *et al.* Dasatinib (BMS-354825) tyrosine kinase inhibitor suppresses invasion and induces cell cycle arrest and apoptosis of head and neck squamous cell carcinoma and non-small cell lung cancer cells. *Clin Cancer Res* 2005;**11**:6924–32.
90. Carducci MA, Musib L, Kies MS, *et al.* Phase I dose escalation and pharmacokinetic study of enzastaurin, an oral protein kinase C beta inhibitor, in patients with advanced cancer. *J Clin Oncol* 2006;**24**:4092–9.
91. Specenier PM, Ciuleanu T, Latz JE, *et al.* Pharmacokinetic evaluation of platinum derived from cisplatin administered alone and with pemetrexed in head and neck cancer patients. *Cancer Chemother Pharmacol* 2009;**64**:233–41.
92. Mazumdar A, Henderson YC, El-Naggar AK, *et al.* Aurora kinase A inhibition and paclitaxel as targeted combination therapy for head and neck squamous cell carcinoma. *Head Neck* 2009;**31**:625–34.
93. Hao Y, Xie T, Korotcov A, *et al.* Salvianolic acid B inhibits growth of head and neck squamous cell carcinoma *in vitro* and *in vivo* via cyclooxygenase-2 and apoptotic pathways. *Int J Cancer* 2009;**124**:2200–9.
94. Allen C, Saigal K, Nottingham L, *et al.* Bortezomib-induced apoptosis with limited clinical response is accompanied by inhibition of canonical but not alternative nuclear factor-{kappa} B subunits in head and neck cancer. *Clin Cancer Res* 2008;**14**:4175–85.
95. Chen Z, Ricker JL, Malhotra PS, *et al.* Differential bortezomib sensitivity in head and neck cancer lines corresponds to proteasome, nuclear factor-kappa B and activator protein-1 related mechanisms. *Mol Cancer Ther* 2008;**7**:1949–60.
96. Li C, Li R, Grandis JR, *et al.* Bortezomib induces apoptosis via Bim and Bik up-regulation and synergizes with cisplatin in the killing of head and neck squamous cell carcinoma cells. *Mol Cancer Ther* 2008;**7**:1647–55.
97. Wagenblast J, Baghi M, Arnoldner C, *et al.* Effect of bortezomib and cetuximab in EGF-stimulated HNSCC. *Anticancer Res* 2008;**28**:2239–43.
98. Gillenwater AM, Zhong M, Lotan R. Histone deacetylase inhibitor suberoylanilide hydroxamic acid induces apoptosis through both mitochondrial and Fas (Cd95) signaling in head and neck squamous carcinoma cells. *Mol Cancer Ther* 2007;**6**:2967–75.
99. Boehm AL, Sen M, Seethala R, *et al.* Combined targeting of epidermal growth factor receptor, signal transducer and activator of transcription-3, and Bcl-X(L) enhances antitumor effects in squamous cell carcinoma of the head and neck. *Mol Pharmacol* 2008;**73**: 1632–42.
100. Xi S, Gooding WE, Grandis JR. *In vivo* anti-tumor efficacy of STAT3 blockade using a transcription factor decoy approach: Implications for cancer therapy. *Oncogene* 2005;**24**:970–9.
101. Leong PL, Andrews GA, Johnson DE, *et al.* Targeted inhibition of Stat3 with a decoy oligonucleotide abrogates head and neck cancer cell growth. *Proc Natl Acad Sci USA* 2003;**100**: 4138–43.
102. Herrero R, Castellsagué X, Pawlita M, *et al.* IARC Multicenter Oral Cancer Study Group. *J Natl Cancer Inst* 2003;**95**:1772–83.
103. Lo WY, Lai CC, Hua CH, *et al.* S100A8 is identified as a biomarker of HPV18-infected oral squamous cell carcinomas by suppression subtraction hybridization, clinical proteomics analysis, and immunohistochemistry staining. *J Proteome Res* 2007;**6**:2143–51.

Potentially Malignant Disorders of the Oral Cavity

David C. Williams and William T. McGaw

The term 'potentially malignant disorder' (PMD) of the oral cavity was created by a working group of the WHO Collaborating Centre for Oral Pathology and Precancer. It is currently used to describe 'white plaques of questionable risk, having excluded other known diseases and diseases that carry no increased risk for cancer' [1]. Not all lesions under the umbrella of PMD transform into cancer, but they are still included as they belong to a morphological group that has an increased potential for malignant transformation [1, 2]. Several clinical entities can be classified as a PMD, with the most common being leukoplakia, erythroplakia, lichen planus, oral submucous fibrosis, palatal lesions in reverse smokers, actinic keratosis and hereditary disorders with increased risk [1]. This chapter will examine oral leukoplakia, oral lichen planus (OLP), erythroplakia and oral submucous fibrosis; the clinical presentation, prevalence and risk factors, histology, molecular genetics, risk of malignant transformation and treatment will be discussed.

Leukoplakia

Leukoplakia was defined in 1978 as a white patch that carries an increased risk for malignant transformation. Several attempts have been made through international collaboration to further refine the definition and classification of leukoplakia [1]. Through these efforts, leukoplakia is now defined as 'a white plaque of questionable

D.C. Williams (✉)
Division of General Surgery, 2D4.39 Walter Mackenzie Health Sciences Center,
8440-112 Street, Edmonton, AB T6G 2B7, Canada
e-mail: dcw@ualberta.ca

W.T. McGaw
Division of Oral Medicine and Pathology, University of Alberta,
Room 5082, Dentistry-Pharmacy Building, Edmonton, AB T6G 2NA, Canada

© The Author(s) 2012
K.A. Pathak, R.W. Nason (eds.), *Controversies in Oral Cancer*,
Head and Neck Cancer Clinics, DOI 10.1007/978-81-322-2574-4_2

risk, having excluded (other) known diseases or disorders that carry no increased risk for cancer' [1, 2]. White lesions that carry no known potential for malignancy include candidiasis, aspirin burn, frictional lesions, hairy leukoplakia, leukoedema, linea alba, lupus erythematosus, lesions resulting from habitual biting or chewing (morsicatio), papilloma, secondary syphilis, nicotinic stomatitis and white sponge naevus [2].

Clinically, leukoplakia can present as a white patch involving any site in the oral cavity. These lesions can be described as being homogeneous and non-homogeneous. Homogeneous lesions are uniformly white, flat and thin. Non-homogeneous lesions may be either irregularly flat or nodular, and typically have both white and red areas, occasionally termed erythroleukoplakia. A subset of non-homogeneous lesions is verrucous leukoplakia, which is typically uniformly white, but its verrucous nature distinguishes it from homogeneous leukoplakia. A subtype of verrucous leukoplakia is proliferative leukoplakia, which is multifocal and aggressive in its malignant potential [3].

The estimated prevalence is 1 % in males <30 years of age, increasing to 8 % in males >70 years of age. The prevalence in women is lower, with 2 % of women >70 years of age being affected [4].

Risk factors for the development of leukoplakia are either idiopathic or related to tobacco use. The type of tobacco used determines the site in the oral cavity that is affected, with reverse cigar smoking causing lesions on the hard palate, chewing causing a lesion at the site of tobacco placement, and cigarette smoking affecting the buccal mucosa. Lesions tend to regress with discontinuation of tobacco use [5, 6]. Alcohol is probably involved in the development of leukoplakia, but the evidence on the importance of its role is conflicting [6–8]. The impact of human papillomavirus (HPV) infection is also debated. Some studies have shown the importance of HPV infection in the development of leukoplakia, but a recent paper shows a lack of association between HPV infection and leukoplakia, specifically verrucous leukoplakia [9].

The most important indicator for leukoplakia to potentially undergo malignant transformation is the presence of epithelial dysplasia. Leukoplakia can be divided into dysplastic and non-dysplastic varieties [2]. Dysplasia is a histological term that describes varying degrees of abnormal epithelial change [10]. It is a spectrum of changes and can be described as mild, moderate and severe, with severe dysplasia known as carcinoma in situ. Histological changes include an increased nuclear-to-cytoplasmic ratio, increased rate of mitotic figures, cellular pleomorphism and nuclear hyperchromatism. It is important to realize that significant intra-observer variation exists in the interpretation of dysplasia, despite clearly defined histological changes [11]. Keeping this in mind, and also the fact that malignant transformation has been described in non-dysplastic lesions, the presence or absence of dysplasia is not an entirely reliable marker when discussing the risk of malignant transformation with the patient [12]. Other factors that increase the chance of leukoplakia transforming into malignant disease include female gender, long duration of leukoplakia, leukoplakia in non-smokers, location on the tongue and floor of mouth, size >200 mm^3 and non-homogeneous type [2].

The rate of malignant transformation varies from site to site in the oral cavity and between populations worldwide [2]. One observational study looking at four regions in India carried out in the 1960s and 1970s quoted a transformation rate of 0.3 % per year [13]. Higher rates have been identified in nations in the West, with studies suggesting a rate of as high as 8.9 % per year [6, 14]. Many of these differences are attributable to the populations being studied, the varied usage of tobacco and the period of follow up [6]. Petti has calculated a global transformation rate of 1.36 % and has suggested that there should be more cases than currently reported; he proposes that the difference is probably due to under-reporting of the condition in developing countries [15].

Molecular diagnostic techniques are becoming more useful, not only in detecting malignant disease, but in predicting the behaviour of certain lesions [16, 17]. Attempts to localize cytogenetic abnormalities have identified loss of heterozygosity, microsatellite instability, chromosomal abnormality, telomere activity and specific genetic abnormalities, which may predict dysplastic changes and possible malignant transformation [17]. Loss of herterozygosity is a mechanism by which genetic loci containing tumour suppressor genes are eliminated, and can result in a 33-fold increase in the risk of malignant transformation [18]. Microsatellite instability—in which base pairs are inserted or deleted—is seen in 55 % of leukoplastic lesions, and a trend to a higher level of instability is seen in lesions that undergo malignant transformation [17, 19]. Chromosomal aneuploidy has been identified in leukoplastic lesions; it was thought to be an independent risk factor for malignant transformation. The data supporting this have been retracted, and there is no good evidence that aneuploidy is an independent risk factor for malignant transformation [17]. Several studies have identified polysomy in leukoplakia, which shows a tendency for malignant transformation if the area of leukoplakia contains cells with trisomy 9 [20]. Telomeres are tandem repeats of TTAGGG at the end of human chromosomes, which prevent degradation and fusion; they shorten with age [17]. Telomere activity has been found to be higher in leukoplastic lesions and a correlation is seen between telomere activity and dysplastic changes [21]. Tumour suppressor genes have been studied in oral cavity squamous cell carcinoma (SCC) and oral leukoplakia [16, 17]. p53 mutations have been studied extensively and their expression has been identified in 90 % of leukoplakia when this lies outside the normal oral cavity mucosa. Studies have shown that the identification of p53 by immunohistochemistry in oral leukoplakia is correlated with a higher risk of malignant transformation [22]. Many studies have identified mutations and chromosomal abnormalities [16–21]. Work will continue to shed light on these important events, which are at the root of malignant transformation. However, these markers are currently not used widely in the management of a patient with oral leukoplakia.

Given the fact that leukoplakia has a relatively low risk of malignant transformation, together with a lack of good scientific evidence that surgical or medical management of these lesions decreases the risk of transformation, the physician has to decide whether to treat these lesions in the first place. Some patients may have symptoms related to leukoplakia, in which case management is justified. Most patients, however, have no symptoms. On the other hand, because of the relatively low morbidity of surgical management and certain medical management strategies, it seems reasonable to treat this patient population actively. The management algorithm described in the succeeding paragraphs is used at our institution and is similar to that presented in the literature [2].

If a cause for leukoplakia is suggested, the aetiological factor should be discontinued and the patient followed up for 6–8 weeks. This observation period is based purely on experience and does seem to be a reasonable period for observation. If the leukoplakia persists, biopsy should be carried out to determine if there is any evidence of dysplasia and, if so, to what degree. If the lesion is small (<2 cm) an excisional biopsy should be performed. Larger lesions can be managed with representative biopsies. Most biopsies can be conducted under local anaesthesia, but general anaesthesia may have to be considered for larger lesions. If multiple areas of leukoplakia are seen, field mapping of the areas involved can be done under general anaesthesia [2, 23].

Once the diagnosis of leukoplakia has been confirmed, it should be decided whether to treat or to observe the lesion. Observation, with frequent visits to the clinic, photography and repeat biopsy (if changes are noted) has been advocated by some clinicians. A retrospective study looking at conservative management compared with active treatment, either surgical or medical, showed no difference in the malignant transformation rate [24]. There may be a selection bias, however, in that a lesion deemed to be a lower risk on clinical grounds alone may have been observed, whereas a more aggressive-appearing lesion may have undergone treatment [25].

Treatment primarily involves surgical techniques, as medical options (discussed later) are not effective in preventing malignant transformation of oral leukoplakia [25]. Nevertheless, surgical management of leukoplakia as a means of preventing malignant transformation remains unproven, although it remains a relatively safe and attractive method of treating these lesions [2, 25]. Surgical management includes scalpel excision, laser surgery or cryosurgery. Cryosurgery was popular in the 1970s and 1980s, but has fallen out of favour in most clinical practices [25, 26]. CO_2 lasers can be used to either excise or vaporize the lesion. It is thought that laser use results in less postoperative oedema and pain, and perhaps in less scar contracture [25, 27]. Laser vaporization has the disadvantage of tissue being evaporated and rendering formal histological examination of the specimen impossible. Scalpel excision or the use of a laser as a knife for excision of the lesion has the advantage that formal histological examination of the material is possible. However, the laser may be a preferable option, as it can result in better haemostasis and the depth of tissue injury is less compared with traditional scalpel excision with electrocauterization of bleeding points [27].

An area of homogeneous leukoplakia showing no dysplasia should be excised if it is <2 cm. In most circumstances, excision would be carried out at the initial biopsy. If the lesion is >2 cm and is homogeneous, observation after appropriate representative biopsy is likely, but laser evaporation could be considered. Our centre tends to follow up these patients with observation and photography every 6 months, and biopsy is repeated if any changes are noted on follow up. If the lesion is non-homogeneous, i.e. with an area of erythroleukoplakia, surgical management with scalpel or laser excision, irrespective of the size of the lesion, is undertaken in view of the higher rate of underlying dysplasia and presumed malignant transformation [2]. Scalpel excision is preferable so that appropriate histological examination can be carried out. Verrucous leukoplakia should be excised, if possible, but if the extent is too large, laser evaporation could be considered after appropriate biopsy.

Non-surgical or medical management of leukoplakia, other than observation, has been suggested as a viable treatment option, given its ease of application and its potential cost-saving benefits. Medical options include carotenoids, vitamin A, bleomycin and mixed teas. Studies examining non-surgical options have been extensively reviewed in a Cochrane collaboration review [28]. Agents examined included systemic beta-carotene, systemic vitamin A and retinoids, lycopene, local ketorolac and mixed tea applied locally as well as ingested. None of the systemic treatments were found to be superior to placebo in preventing malignant transformation of leukoplakia. When clinical resolution was examined, benefit was seen for beta-carotene or lycopene administered systemically when compared to controls. Vitamin A and retinoids showed a significant but small advantage when compared with controls. Discontinuation of therapy resulted in a high rate of relapse. In addition, adverse side-effects, including pain, oral erosions, dryness, facial oedema and headache were reported in 100 % of the patients. The authors of the Cochrane review have concluded that none of the non-surgical options were found to be effective in preventing malignant transformation, and if the options were effective in healing the leukoplakia, the relapse rate appears to be higher [28–33]. The use of photodynamic therapy has been examined in the treatment of oral leukoplakia; complete regression has been observed in verrucous lesions [34, 35]. However, the few numbers of patients enrolled in studies and short follow-up periods of observation do not allow this method of treatment to be recommended as a standard of care [36, 37].

Oral Lichen Planus

Lichen planus is a relatively common inflammatory mucocutaneous disease, with a prevalence of 0.1–4 %, depending on the population sampled. It is generally a disease of middle-aged and elderly people; the female-to-male ratio is ~2:1. Intraoral manifestations of lichen planus are very common and they may precede or coexist with skin lesions. In some instances they may be the exclusive manifestations of the disease. Compared with skin lesions, the lesions of OLP are far more chronic [38, 40–42].

Oral lichen planus can involve any site of the oral mucosa, but is most commonly seen as bilateral lesions involving the buccal mucosa, gingiva and lateral borders of the tongue. The floor of the mouth is the least commonly affected. Clinically, a variety of presentations of OLP are seen [43–45]. The reticular form of OLP is usually asymptomatic and can present as a white, linear, annular or lacy pattern, commonly seen on the buccal mucosa, lips, tongue or gingiva. OLP may present as white angular papules and plaques, often on the dorsum of the tongue or buccal mucosa, and can appear as a non-specific white lesion. The plaques can be multiple and are usually associated with reticular white lesions, with or without atrophic or erosive lesions. Erosive forms of OLP may present with erythema caused by inflammation and/or epithelial thinning, together with ulceration and pseudomembrane formation. Frequently, the erosive form of OLP presents with white striations at the periphery of the erosions and is often associated with burning pain and sensitivity. Although OLP is frequently asymptomatic, the atrophic/erosive form can cause symptoms ranging from a burning sensation to severe pain and often requires treatment.

In OLP, the majority of T-cells within the epithelium and adjacent to the damaged basal keratinocytes are activated CD8+ (cytotoxic) lymphocytes. Most of the T-cells in the subjacent lamina propria are CD4+ (helper) lymphocytes. The antigen triggering these T-cells may be a self-peptide, thus defining lichen planus as a true autoimmune disease, or it may be exogenous [46, 47]. Activated CD8+ (cytotoxic) T-cells trigger keratinocyte apoptosis through mechanisms that may involve tumour necrosis factor-alpha or granzyme B. In cases in which this is the predominant inflammatory event, the clinical appearance is that of an atrophic or eroded lesion. In contrast, white lesions of OLP reflect zones of keratinocyte hyperproliferation, which may result from the activation of the inflammatory mediator nuclear factor kappa B and the inhibition of the transforming growth factor control pathway (TGF-beta/smad) [41, 42, 48, 49].

Most cases of OLP are idiopathic. However, a subset of cases may be attributed to identifiable factors. When drugs or dental materials induce lesions similar to OLP, the term 'oral lichenoid reaction' is generally used [50]. The drugs most commonly implicated in oral lichenoid reactions are the non-steroidal anti-inflammatory medications and angiotensin-converting enzyme inhibitors. Other drugs known to cause lichenoid eruptions include thiazides, penicillamine, beta-blockers, oral hypoglycaemics, phenothiazines, carbamazepine, allopurinol, gold salts, lithium and many others [39, 51–54]. The most reliable method of diagnosing lichenoid drug reactions is to see if the reaction resolves after the drug has been withdrawn, and if it returns when the drug is taken again [39]. In a small subset of patients, lesions resembling OLP may occur in direct relation to amalgam restorations, and these oral lesions may improve after substitution of the amalgam by other materials. Unfortunately, other dental restorative materials, including gold alloys, have also been associated with such lichenoid contact reactions, albeit rarely [55, 56].

The psychological profile of the OLP patient should also be taken into account. Studies have reported higher levels of anxiety, greater depression and increased incidence of psychiatric disorders in OLP patients compared with a control group; stress is one of the most frequently reported causes of acute exacerbations of OLP [57, 58].

The involvement of viral agents in OLP has been suggested, but any causal role remains speculative. Viral antigens might be expressed on the affected keratinocyte surface membrane, just as are the human major histocompatibility antigens. Viruses for which an association with OLP has been suggested anecdotally include varicella zoster virus, Epstein–Barr virus, cytomegalovirus, human herpes virus 6 and HPV [39, 50]. Since the first report in 1991, more than 80 papers worldwide, including numerous controlled studies, have suggested an association between OLP and hepatitis C virus (HCV) infection [39, 59]. A systematic review demonstrated that a significantly higher proportion of HCV seropositivity was documented in patients with OLP, with an odds ratio of 5.7 [60]. Conversely, in HCV-positive patients, the estimated prevalence of OLP is significantly higher than that expected in the respective geographical areas [61, 62]. However, geographical discrepancies exist, and while the association between OLP and HCV seropositivity has been well documented in populations from the Mediterranean, Asia and the USA, this association could not be demonstrated in France or the United Kingdom [50].

The putative pathogenic link between OLP and HCV is still under investigation. While it has been hypothesized that HCV might share common epitopes with host keratinocytes, studies have failed to demonstrate this. It is therefore more likely that the pathogenic immune response occurring in OLP lesions in these patients targets epithelial cells expressing HCV antigens [51, 65]. In this regard, several groups have reported detecting HCV RNA in the epithelial cells in patients with HCV [64].

Because only 20–30 % of HCV-infected individuals develop clinically evident acute hepatitis, it is likely that at least some patients with OLP are unaware that they have HCV. This suggests that consideration should perhaps be given to screening patients with OLP for HCV, particularly in geographical regions where HCV prevalence is high or if the patient has a history of risk factors for HCV [41, 65].

Available treatment for OLP is not curative and many of them have potentially significant side-effects. Therefore, the objectives of OLP management are to alleviate symptoms in the long term and to prevent and screen for malignant transformation [39, 42, 50].

Patients with reticular and other asymptomatic OLP lesions usually require no active treatment. However, mechanical irritants, such as rough dental restorations or ill-fitting dentures should be addressed, because they may exacerbate OLP lesions by a Koebner phenomenon. In addition, depending on the distribution of lesions, possible lichenoid contact reaction to dental restorative material should be considered. An optimal programme of oral hygiene should be instituted, particularly in patients with gingival OLP [42, 50].

Whenever drug-induced oral lichenoid lesions are suspected, the drug should be withdrawn. However, it may be months before the lesions resolve, so that empirical withdrawal of the drug in question, and its substitution with another, may be warranted [42].

Various treatment regimens have been designed to improve management of symptomatic OLP, including topical agents and systemic therapy. Super-potent topical corticosteroids, such as 0.05 % clobetasole or 0.1 % fluocinonide, remain the mainstay of treatment. The reported complete remission rate of OLP with 0.05 % clobetasole is 47–75 % [50]. Although there are some reports of systemic absorption and adrenal suppression from super-potent topical corticosteroids in the treatment of chronic skin disorders, adrenal suppression has not been found following long-term oral application of these agents [50, 66].

Superimposed *Candida albicans* is present in ~37 % of OLP lesions. Acute exacerbation of candidiasis is the only common side-effect from topical corticosteroid therapy. This can be prevented by having the patient rinse with mycelex or chlorhexidine mouthwashes [40, 67, 68].

Evidence that topical retinoids are more effective than topical corticosteroids in the treatment of OLP is not convincing; they have been associated with adverse effects, such as dryness and desquamation. Whereas topical retinoids may eliminate rapidly the predominantly hyperkeratotic white lesions of OLP, relapse is typically 2–5 weeks after discontinuation of treatment [50, 51, 69].

Calcineurin inhibitors, such as cyclosporin and tacrolimus, interfere with the generation of proinflammatory cytokines by T-lymphocytes and have been used in the treatment of OLP. Cyclosporin has been used as a mouth rinse for treating OLP. However, it is expensive and has been shown to be less effective than topical clobetasole in inducing clinical improvement [42, 70, 71]. At a given concentration, tacrolimus is up to 100 times more powerful than cyclosporin. Efficacy of tacrolimus 0.1 % ointment has been reported in cases of OLP refractory to topical corticosteroids, although some patients have noted flare-ups soon after stopping treatment [50, 51, 72, 73].

The relegation of topical tacrolimus for use in refractory OLP relates to concerns regarding potential carcinogenesis. Tacrolimus 0.1 % was the suspected causative agent of oral SCC of the tongue in a 56-year-old woman who was being treated for OLP [74]. The oral carcinoma developed after 3 years of topical tacrolimus therapy and 6 years after the diagnosis of OLP. Animal studies also suggest that tacrolimus may be a promoter or accelerator of mucocutaneous carcinogenesis and, in 2006, the FDA approved the inclusion of a potential risk of cancer in the labelling of topical tacrolimus, and stated that this agent should be used as second-line therapy [75].

Systemic corticosteroids may be indicated in patients whose condition is unresponsive to topical corticosteroids, particularly if the lesions are widespread. However, adverse effects are possible even on short courses. Systemic corticosteroids should be reserved for severe refractory flare-ups [50, 51]. Systemic retinoids have been used successfully in severe erosive OLP refractory to conventional therapies, but relapses generally occur within 2 months after the drug is stopped. Because of low remission rates, as well as significant side-effects when used systemically, the primary use of retinoids in the management of OLP is discouraged [51, 76].

Azathioprine is used commonly in the treatment of severe recalcitrant cases of OLP. However, the potential for bone marrow suppression or an increased risk of internal malignancies dictates caution in its use [77].

Since the first report in 1910 of a gingival cancer diagnosed in a patient with OLP [78], numerous studies have attempted to address the issue of malignant transformation of OLP. Most of these cases have been analysed by two independent groups of researchers adopting the same criteria [79, 80]. While the best way to establish the putative pre-malignant nature of OLP would be a prospective follow-up study of a group of affected patients and a group of unaffected individuals, including smokers and non-smokers, such a study is not available. Therefore, the best evidence currently available on the potentially pre-malignant nature of OLP is from follow-up studies and retrospective incidence studies [51]. In the earlier published studies, the frequency of malignant transformation ranged from 0 to 12.5 % [2, 41].

Unfortunately, many of these studies lacked clinicopathological correlation in the diagnosis of OLP. In 1978, Krutchkoff et al. recommended strict criteria be adopted to accept definitively the malignant transformation of OLP [79]. After applying these new criteria, they concluded that only 15 of the 223 cases reported in the older literature could be unquestionably accepted as malignant transformation in OLP. The remaining cases were excluded for at least one of the following reasons: Insufficient data to support the diagnosis of OLP appearance of oral cancer in an area anatomically distant from the OLP, and inadequate historical data on previous exposure to carcinogens. More recent reviews, which have adhered to these new criteria, have concluded that the transformation rate probably should be considered to be ~0.5–3 % [81–83].

The reasons for malignant transformation in OLP lesions are not clear. OLP has a higher rate of cell turnover, which may increase the risk of genetic errors. If exposed to a carcinogen, OLP may undergo molecular changes leading to dysplasia and increased cancer risk. However, in the published follow-up studies, smoking and alcohol were certainly not reported to be consistent risk factors, so other factors should be considered [42, 43]. Studies have identified genetic changes in dysplastic OLP which commonly occur in carcinogenesis. It has been proposed that the genetic instability of OLP can be induced by the repetitive process of destruction and proliferation of basal epithelial cells and is associated with dysplasia [84, 85].

A possible role for microbial factors has been suggested. One factor may be *Candida albicans,* as this has been associated with malignant development in some leukoplastic lesions, and such yeasts have been identified in OLP [86]. Another possibility is that herpes simplex virus or HPV are involved, both of which have been implicated as risk factors in carcinogenesis and are found in OLP [87].

Finally, in considering possible factors contributing to malignant transformation in OLP, one can look at the impact of the actual OLP treatments themselves. Patients affected by OLP are often subjected to medical treatments for long periods. The drugs of first choice are immunosuppressive agents, such as corticosteroids, tacrolimus, cyclosporin and azathioprine. Theoretically, immunosuppressive agents could trigger or predispose to malignant transformation. For example, cyclosporin can promote cancer progression, both by a direct cellular effect and by an effect on the host's immune cells. Concern has also been expressed regarding topical tacrolimus, which is a common treatment for the management of refractory lesions of OLP [74, 75, 88].

As to the type of OLP most likely to undergo malignant change, several authors have reported atrophic, ulcerative and erosive OLP lesions as the lesions with the greatest preponderance for malignant development. Further, in some of the studies, location preponderance was revealed, with most carcinomas developing in the tongue, gingival mucosa or buccal mucosa [39, 44, 51, 89].

In the case of lesions of OLP that initially demonstrate no features of dysplasia on biopsy, it would be desirable to be able to identify the subset of lesions that are at increased risk for future malignant transformation. However, whereas the identification of markers of high-risk lesions has been extensively investigated in leukoplakia, investigative techniques, such as DNA content or loss of heterozygosity, have been tested to date in OLP lesions only to a very limited extent [84, 90, 91].

All OLP patients should avoid tobacco and alcohol and should be monitored for potential malignant transformation. Empirically, follow up has been recommended twice yearly for erosive cases and annually for hyperkeratotic cases. However, the most appropriate frequency of clinical screening is not yet established [82].

Erythroplakia

Erythroplakia was defined as 'any lesion of the oral mucosa that presents as bright red velvety plaques which cannot be characterized clinically or pathologically as any other recognizable condition' [92, 93]. The definition was further refined in 1997 as a 'fiery red patch that cannot be characterized clinically or pathologically as any other definable condition', a definition that is now widely accepted [94].

Little is known about the prevalence of erythroplakia, as cases were not published until the 1980s, and the published studies are all from South and Southeast Asia. The published data suggest a prevalence rate between 0.02 and 0.83 % [92].

Clinically, erythroplakia appears as a soft, velvety, flat or depressed lesion. The surface is smooth or granular [2]. A well-defined margin adjacent to normal mucosa may be present [94]. Typically, lesions are solitary and do not cover extensive areas of the oral cavity, a fact that can be used to distinguish erythroplakia from erosive lichen planus, systemic lupus erythematosus, and erythematous candidiasis [2, 92].

The rate at which men and women are affected is equal; middle-aged and elderly people are at greatest risk of developing erythroleukoplakia [2, 95, 96]. The locations that are most commonly involved include the soft palate, buccal mucosa and the floor of mouth, with lesions typically measuring <1.5 cm [92].

Risk factors for developing erythroplakia are not clearly understood, but alcohol and tobacco are thought to play a major role [92]. Large case–control studies from India showed that chewing tobacco and consuming alcohol were strong risk factors for developing erythroplakia in the Indian population [7, 97]. Betel chewing in the absence of tobacco intake and in non-drinkers was also examined in the same population, and was found to be an independent risk factor for the development of erythroplakia [98]. *Candida albicans* has also been implicated in the pathogenesis of erythroplakia [92].

Cytogenetic abnormalities identified in erythroplakia include DNA ploidy and p53 mutations. Lesions with DNA aneuploidy and those showing mutation in p53 also had a higher rate of malignant transformation [99, 100].

Erythroplakia is a clinical term and the histopathological changes seen in the clinical lesion are related to dysplasia. Dysplasia describes the degree of abnormal epithelial changes, including an increased nuclear-to-cytoplasmic ratio, increased rate of mitotic figures, cellular pleomorphism and nuclear hyperchromatism [10]. Dysplasia can be graded on a spectrum from low- to high-grade to carcinoma in situ. Erythroplakia commonly shows at least moderate to severe dysplasia, with one study suggesting that ≤50 % of patients showed invasive carcinoma and 40 % showed carcinoma in situ ($n=58$) [2, 95].

The rate of malignant transformation of erythroplakia is high. Given that severe dysplasia is seen in biopsies of erythroplakia, it can be assumed that these progress to invasive malignancy. A transformation rate varying from 14 to 50 % is quoted in the literature [92].

On account of the high rate of malignant transformation and the fact that erythroplakia is usually symptomatic, treatment of the lesion is mandatory; its excision with scalpel or laser is the treatment of choice [2]. Biopsy and observation are unnecessary if only mild dysplasia is identified, again because of the high rate of malignant transformation. Data on chemoprevention of erythroplakia are lacking in the literature.

Erythroplakia, the true fiery red patch affecting the oral cavity, is a rare condition and published literature on it is scant. It is clear that these lesions have the highest malignant potential of all PMDs. Clinicians should be aware of this fact and, because of the high rate of recurrence, all lesions should be treated surgically with long-term follow up.

Submucous Fibrosis

Oral submucous fibrosis is a PMD that is related to chewing of areca nut and betel leaf. The disease is primarily seen in people of Asian descent and affects the oral cavity, pharynx and upper oesophagus. Areca nut and betel leaf chewing have increased in popularity in India, and consequently so have the number of cases of submucous fibrosis [101, 102]. It is estimated that five million people in India have oral submucous fibrosis [103]. It is noteworthy that ≤20 % of the world's population chews areca to some degree, suggesting that the prevalence of oral submucous fibrosis will probably increase in the coming years [103].

Patients presenting with oral submucous fibrosis typically complain of sores in the mouth and intolerance to spicy foods [103]. The stomatitis progresses to fibrosis. The resulting scar causes stiffening and blanching of the mucosa with progressive trismus. Fibrous bands are seen on the buccal mucosa, the pharyngeal mucosa and around the lips [2].

Multiple studies have amply substantiated the fact that areca nut is the main aetiological factor in oral submucous fibrosis, and acts in a dose-dependent fashion [104]. The areca nut contains alkaloids and tannins that can alter either collagen deposition or degradation, resulting in the obliteration of the lamina propria by fibroblasts [101].

Epithelial dysplasia is seen in oral submucous fibrosis in 10–15 % of the population at risk [101, 105]. The annual malignant transformation rate in India was found to be 6.4 % in 66 patients followed over 17 years, suggesting a high degree of malignant potential of the lesion [106].

The treatment of oral submucous fibrosis primarily involves medical and surgical therapy. Medical therapy in the form of intraluminal injection of corticosteroid has been shown to decrease the amount of contracture. Trismus may be relieved with surgical division of masticatory muscles with the addition of a coronoidectomy

[103]. Given the high rate of malignant transformation seen in these patients, constant vigilance is mandatory and any suspicious lesion must be biopsied. It is important to note that areca nut chewing is increasing in geographical areas where the habit has not been practised traditionally, and the clinician must keep this in mind while making a diagnosis, and also understand the risk of malignant transformation [103].

References

1. Warnakulasuriya S, Johnson NW, van der Waal I. Nomenclature and classification of potentially malignant disorders of the oral mucosa. *J Oral Pathol Med* 2007;**36**:575–80.
2. van der Waal I. Potentially malignant disorders of the oral and oropharyngeal mucosa: Terminology, classification and present concepts of management. *Oral Oncol* 2009;**45**: 317–23.
3. van der Waal I. Potentially malignant disorders of the oral and oropharyngeal mucosa: Present concepts of management. *Oral Oncol* 2010;**46**:423–5.
4. Ribeiro AS, Salles PR, da Silva TA, *et al.* A review of the non-surgical treatment of oral leukoplakia. *Int J Dent* 2010;**2010**:186018.
5. Roed-Petersen B. Effect on oral leukoplakia of reducing or ceasing tobacco smoking. *Acta Derm Venereol* 1982;**62**:164–7.
6. Napier SS, Speight PM. Natural history of potentially malignant oral lesions and conditions: An overview of the literature. *J Oral Pathol Med* 2008;**37**:1–10.
7. Hashibe M, Jacob BJ, Thomas G, *et al.* Socioeconomic status, lifestyle factors and oral premalignant lesions. *Oral Oncol* 2003;**39**:664–71.
8. Dietrich T, Reichart PA, Scheifele C. Clinical risk factors of oral leukoplakia in a representative sample of the US population. *Oral Oncol* 2004;**40**:158–63.
9. Bagan JV, Jimenez Y, Murillo J, *et al.* Lack of association between proliferative verrucous leukoplakia and human papillomavirus infection. *J Oral Maxillofac Surg* 2007;**65**: 46–9.
10. Eugene N. SJ (ed). *Cancer of the head and neck.* 3rd ed. Philadelphia: WWB, Saunders; 1996.
11. Kujan O, Khattab A, Oliver RJ, *et al.* Why oral histopathology suffers inter-observer variability on grading oral epithelial dysplasia: An attempt to understand the sources of variation. *Oral Oncol* 2007;**43**:224–31.
12. Holmstrup P, Vedtofte P, Reibel J, *et al.* Long-term treatment outcome of oral premalignant lesions. *Oral Oncol* 2006;**42**:461–74.
13. Gupta PC, Mehta FS, Daftary DK, *et al.* Incidence rates of oral cancer and natural history of oral precancerous lesions in a 10-year follow-up study of Indian villagers. *Community Dent Oral Epidemiol* 1980;**8**:283–333.
14. Lind PO. Malignant transformation in oral leukoplakia. *Scand J Dent Res* 1987;**95**:449–55.
15. Petti S. Pooled estimate of world leukoplakia prevalence: A systematic review. *Oral Oncol* 2003;**39**:770–80.
16. Bilodeau E, Alawi F, Costello BJ, *et al.* Molecular diagnostics for head and neck pathology. *Oral Maxillofac Surg Clin North Am* 2010;**22**:183–94.
17. Mithani SK, Mydlarz WK, Grumbine FL, *et al.* Molecular genetics of premalignant oral lesions. *Oral Dis* 2007;**13**:126–33.
18. Rosin MP, Cheng X, Poh C, *et al.* Use of allelic loss to predict malignant risk for low-grade oral epithelial dysplasia. *Clin Cancer Res* 2000;**6**:357–62.
19. Partridge M, Emilion G, Pateromichelakis S, *et al.* Allelic imbalance at chromosomal loci implicated in the pathogenesis of oral precancer, cumulative loss and its relationship with progression to cancer. *Oral Oncol* 1998;**34**:77–83.
20. Lee JS, Kim SY, Hong WK, *et al.* Detection of chromosomal polysomy in oral leukoplakia, a premalignant lesion. *J Natl Cancer Inst* 1993;**85**:1951–4.

21. Fujimoto R, Kamata N, Yokoyama K, et al. Expression of telomerase components in oral keratinocytes and squamous cell carcinomas. *Oral Oncol* 2001;**37**:132–40.
22. Kovesi G, Szende B. Changes in apoptosis and mitotic index, p53 and Ki67 expression in various types of oral leukoplakia. *Oncology* 2003;**65**:331–6.
23. Thomson PJ, Hamadah O. Cancerisation within the oral cavity: The use of 'field mapping biopsies' in clinical management. *Oral Oncol* 2007;**43**:20–6.
24. Schepman KP, Bezemer PD, van der Meij EH, et al. Tobacco usage in relation to the anatomical site of oral leukoplakia. *Oral Dis* 2001;**7**:25–7.
25. Lodi G, Porter S. Management of potentially malignant disorders: Evidence and critique. *J Oral Pathol Med* 2008;**37**:63–9.
26. Sako K, Marchetta FC, Hayes RL. Cryotherapy of intraoral leukoplakia. *Am J Surg* 1972;**124**:482–4.
27. Meltzer C. Surgical management of oral and mucosal dysplasias: The case for laser excision. *J Oral Maxillofac Surg* 2007;**65**:293–5.
28. Lodi G, Sardella A, Bez C, et al. Interventions for treating oral leukoplakia. *Cochrane Database Syst Rev* 2006;**4**:CD001829.
29. Stich HF, Hornby AP, Mathew B, et al. Response of oral leukoplakias to the administration of vitamin A. *Cancer Lett* 1988;**40**:93–101.
30. Sankaranarayanan R, Mathew B, Varghese C, et al. Chemoprevention of oral leukoplakia with vitamin A and beta carotene: An assessment. *Oral Oncol* 1997;**33**:231–6.
31. Piattelli A, Fioroni M, Santinelli A, et al. Bcl-2 expression and apoptotic bodies in 13-cis-retinoic acid (isotretinoin)-topically treated oral leukoplakia: A pilot study. *Oral Oncol* 1999;**35**:314–20.
32. Hong WK, Endicott J, Itri LM, et al. 13-cis-retinoic acid in the treatment of oral leukoplakia. *N Engl J Med* 1986;**315**:1501–5.
33. Gaeta GM, Gombos F, Femiano F, et al. Acitretin and treatment of the oral leucoplakias. A model to have an active molecules release. *J Eur Acad Dermatol Venereol* 2000;**14**: 473–8.
34. Fan KF, Hopper C, Speight PM, et al. Photodynamic therapy using 5-aminolevulinic acid for premalignant and malignant lesions of the oral cavity. *Cancer* 1996;**78**:1374–83.
35. Chen HM, Yu CH, Tu PC, et al. Successful treatment of oral verrucous hyperplasia and oral leukoplakia with topical 5-aminolevulinic acid-mediated photodynamic therapy. *Lasers Surg Med* 2005;**37**:114–22.
36. Sieron A, Adamek M, Kawczyk-Krupka A, et al. Photodynamic therapy (PDT) using topically applied delta-aminolevulinic acid (ALA) for the treatment of oral leukoplakia. *J Oral Pathol Med* 2003;**32**:330–6.
37. Kubler A, Haase T, Rheinwald M, et al. Treatment of oral leukoplakia by topical application of 5-aminolevulinic acid. *Int J Oral Maxillofac Surg* 1998;**27**:466–9.
38. Bouquot JE. Common oral lesions found during a mass screening examination. *J Am Dent Assoc* 1986;**112**:50–7.
39. Scully C, Beyli M, Ferreiro MC, et al. Update on oral lichen planus: Etiopathogenesis and management. *Crit Rev Oral Biol Med* 1998;**9**:86–122.
40. Markopoulos A, Kayavis I, Paleologoy A, et al. Oral lichen planus. A clinical study of 228 cases. *Hell Stomatol Chron* 1989;**33**:107–11.
41. Lodi G, Scully C, Carrozzo M, et al. Current controversies in oral lichen planus: Report of an international consensus meeting. Part 1. Viral infections and etiopathogenesis. *Oral Surg Oral Med Oral Pathol Oral Radiol Endod* 2005;**100**:40–51.
42. Scully C, Carrozzo M. Oral mucosal disease: Lichen planus. *Br J Oral Maxillofac Surg* 2008;**46**:15–21.
43. Epstein JB, Wan LS, Gorsky M, et al. Oral lichen planus: Progress in understanding its malignant potential and the implications for clinical management. *Oral Surg Oral Med Oral Pathol Oral Radiol Endod* 2003;**96**:32–7.

44. Silverman S Jr, Gorsky M, Lozada-Nur F. A prospective follow-up study of 570 patients with oral lichen planus: Persistence, remission, and malignant association. *Oral Surg Oral Med Oral Pathol* 1985;**60**:30–4.
45. Gorsky M, Raviv M, Moskona D, *et al.* Clinical characteristics and treatment of patients with oral lichen planus in Israel. *Oral Surg Oral Med Oral Pathol Oral Radiol Endod* 1996;**82**: 644–9.
46. Kilpi AM. Activation marker analysis of mononuclear cell infiltrates of oral lichen planus *in situ. Scand J Dent Res* 1987;**95**:174–80.
47. Jungell P, Konttinen YT, Nortamo P, *et al.* Immunoelectron microscopic study of distribution of T-cell subsets in oral lichen planus. *Scand J Dent Res* 1989;**97**:361–7.
48. Santoro A, Majorana A, Bardellini E, *et al.* NF-kappaB expression in oral and cutaneous lichen planus. *J Pathol* 2003;**201**:466–72.
49. Karatsaidis A, Schreurs O, Axell T, *et al.* Inhibition of the transforming growth factor-beta/ Smad signaling pathway in the epithelium of oral lichen. *J Invest Dermatol* 2003;**121**: 1283–90.
50. Farhi D, Dupin N. Pathophysiology, etiologic factors, and clinical management of oral lichen planus, part I: Facts and controversies. *Clin Dermatol* 2010;**28**:100–8.
51. Lodi G, Scully C, Carrozzo M, *et al.* Current controversies in oral lichen planus: Report of an international consensus meeting. Part 2. Clinical management and malignant transformation. *Oral Surg Oral Med Oral Pathol Oral Radiol Endod* 2005;**100**:164–78.
52. Potts AJ, Hamburger J, Scully C. The medication of patients with oral lichen planus and the association of nonsteroidal anti-inflammatory drugs with erosive lesions. *Oral Surg Oral Med Oral Pathol* 1987;**64**:541–3.
53. Firth NA, Reade PC. Angiotensin-converting enzyme inhibitors implicated in oral mucosal lichenoid reactions. *Oral Surg Oral Med Oral Pathol* 1989;**67**:41–4.
54. Robertson WD, Wray D. Ingestion of medication among patients with oral keratoses including lichen planus. *Oral Surg Oral Med Oral Pathol* 1992;**74**:183–5.
55. Smart ER, Macleod RI, Lawrence CM. Resolution of lichen planus following removal of amalgam restorations in patients with proven allergy to mercury salts: A pilot study. *Br Dent J* 1995;**178**:108–12.
56. Laeijendecker R, van Joost T. Oral manifestations of gold allergy. *J Am Acad Dermatol* 1994;**30**:205–9.
57. Rojo-Moreno JL, Bagan JV, Rojo-Moreno J, *et al.* Psychologic factors and oral lichen planus. A psychometric evaluation of 100 cases. *Oral Surg Oral Med Oral Pathol Oral Radiol Endod* 1998;**86**:687–91.
58. McCartan BE. Psychological factors associated with oral lichen planus. *J Oral Pathol Med* 1995;**24**:273–5.
59. Rebora A. Lichen planus and the liver. *Lancet* 1981;**2**:805–6.
60. Lodi G, Giuliani M, Majorana A, *et al.* Lichen planus and hepatitis C virus: A multicentre study of patients with oral lesions and a systematic review. *Br J Dermatol* 2004;**151**: 1172–81.
61. Grote M, Reichart PA, Berg T, *et al.* Hepatitis C virus (HCV) infection and oral lichen planus. *J Hepatol* 1998;**29**:1034–5.
62. Henderson L, Muir M, Mills PR, *et al.* Oral health of patients with hepatitis C virus infection: A pilot study. *Oral Dis* 2001;**7**:271–5.
63. Lodi G, Olsen I, Piatelli A, *et al.* Antibodies to epithelial components in oral lichen planus (OLP) associated with hepatitis C virus (HCV) infection. *J Oral Pathol Med* 1997;**26**:36–9.
64. Arrieta JJ, Rodriguez-Inigo E, Casqueiro M, *et al.* Detection of hepatitis C virus replication by in situ hybridization in epithelial cells of anti-hepatitis C virus-positive patients with and without oral lichen planus. *Hepatology* 2000;**32**:97–103.
65. Bigby M. The relationship between lichen planus and hepatitis C clarified. *Arch Dermatol* 2009;**145**:1048–50.

66. Plemons JM, Rees TD, Zachariah NY. Absorption of a topical steroid and evaluation of adrenal suppression in patients with erosive lichen planus. *Oral Surg Oral Med Oral Pathol* 1990;**69**:688–93.
67. Hatchuel DA, Peters E, Lemmer J, *et al.* Candidal infection in oral lichen planus. *Oral Surg Oral Med Oral Pathol* 1990;**70**:172–5.
68. Carbone M, Conrotto D, Carrozzo M, *et al.* Topical corticosteroids in association with miconazole and chlorhexidine in the long-term management of atrophic-erosive oral lichen planus: A placebo-controlled and comparative study between clobetasol and fluocinonide. *Oral Dis* 1999;**5**:44–9.
69. Zegarelli DJ. Treatment of oral lichen planus with topical vitamin A acid. *J Oral Med* 1984;**39**:186–91.
70. Al Johani KA, Hegarty AM, Porter SR, *et al.* Calcineurin inhibitors in oral medicine. *J Am Acad Dermatol* 2009;**61**:829–40.
71. Conrotto D, Carbone M, Carrozzo M, *et al.* Ciclosporin vs. clobetasol in the topical management of atrophic and erosive oral lichen planus: A double-blind, randomized controlled trial. *Br J Dermatol* 2006;**154**:139–45.
72. Rozycki TW, Rogers RS 3rd, Pittelkow MR, *et al.* Topical tacrolimus in the treatment of symptomatic oral lichen planus: A series of 13 patients. *J Am Acad Dermatol* 2002;**46**:27–34.
73. Morrison L, Kratochvil FJ 3rd, Gorman A. An open trial of topical tacrolimus for erosive oral lichen planus. *J Am Acad Dermatol* 2002;**47**:617–20.
74. Becker JC, Houben R, Vetter CS, *et al.* The carcinogenic potential of tacrolimus ointment beyond immune suppression: A hypothesis creating case report. *BMC Cancer* 2006;**6**:7.
75. Niwa Y, Terashima T, Sumi H. Topical application of the immunosuppressant tacrolimus accelerates carcinogenesis in mouse skin. *Br J Dermatol* 2003;**149**:960–7.
76. Woo TY. Systemic isotretinoin treatment of oral and cutaneous lichen planus. *Cutis* 1985;**35**: 385–6, 390–1, 393.
77. Lear JT, English JS. Erosive and generalized lichen planus responsive to azathioprine. *Clin Exp Dermatol* 1996;**21**:56–7.
78. Hallopeau H. Sur un cas de lichen de Wilson gingival avec neoplasie voisine dans la region maxillaire. *Bull Soc Fr Dermatol Syphiligr* 1910;**17**:32.
79. Krutchkoff DJ, Cutler L, Laskowski S. Oral lichen planus: The evidence regarding potential malignant transformation. *J Oral Pathol* 1978;**7**:1–7.
80. Van der Meij EH, Schepman KP, van der Wal JE, *et al.* A review of the recent literature regarding malignant transformation of oral lichen planus. *Oral Surg Oral Med Oral Pathol Oral Radiol Endod* 1999;**88**:307–10.
81. Gonzalez-Moles MA, Scully C, Gil-Montoya JA. Oral lichen planus: Controversies surrounding malignant transformation. *Oral Dis* 2008;**14**:229–43.
82. Mattsson U, Jontell M, Holmstrup P. Oral lichen planus and malignant transformation: Is a recall of patients justified? *Crit Rev Oral Biol Med* 2002;**13**:390–6.
83. Gandolfo S, Richiardi L, Carrozzo M, *et al.* Risk of oral squamous cell carcinoma in 402 patients with oral lichen planus: A follow-up study in an Italian population. *Oral Oncol* 2004;**40**:77–83.
84. Zhang L, Cheng X, Li Y, *et al.* High frequency of allelic loss in dysplastic lichenoid lesions. *Lab Invest* 2000;**80**:233–7.
85. Kim J, Yook JI, Lee EH, *et al.* Evaluation of premalignant potential in oral lichen planus using interphase cytogenetics. *J Oral Pathol Med* 2001;**30**:65–72.
86. Krogh P, Holmstrup P, Thorn JJ, *et al.* Yeast species and biotypes associated with oral leukoplakia and lichen planus. *Oral Surg Oral Med Oral Pathol* 1987;**63**:48–54.
87. Cox M, Maitland N, Scully C. Human herpes simplex-1 and papillomavirus type 16 homologous DNA sequences in normal, potentially malignant and malignant oral mucosa. *Eur J Cancer B Oral Oncol* 1993;**29B**:215–19.
88. Hojo M, Morimoto T, Maluccio M, *et al.* Cyclosporine induces cancer progression by a cell-autonomous mechanism. *Nature* 1999;**397**:530–4.

89. Barnard NA, Scully C, Eveson JW, *et al.* Oral cancer development in patients with oral lichen planus. *J Oral Pathol Med* 1993;**22**:421–4.
90. Sudbo J, Ried T, Bryne M, *et al.* Abnormal DNA content predicts the occurrence of carcinomas in non-dysplastic oral white patches. *Oral Oncol* 2001;**37**:558–65.
91. Zhang L, Michelsen C, Cheng X, *et al.* Molecular analysis of oral lichen planus. A premalignant lesion? *Am J Pathol* 1997;**151**:323–7.
92. Reichart PA, Philipsen HP. Oral erythroplakia—a review. *Oral Oncol* 2005;**41**:551–61.
93. Kramer IR, Lucas RB, Pindborg JJ, *et al.* Definition of leukoplakia and related lesions: An aid to studies on oral precancer. *Oral Surg Oral Med Oral Pathol* 1978;**46**:518–39.
94. Pindborg JJ, Reichart PA, Smith CJ, van der Waal I, in collaboaration with Sobin L.H. and pathologists in 9 countries editors. *Histological typing of cancer and precancer of the oral mucosa.* 2nd ed. Berlin, New York, Tokyo: Springer Verlag; 1997.
95. Shafer WG, Waldron CA. Erythroplakia of the oral cavity. *Cancer* 1975;**36**:1021–8.
96. Hashibe M, Mathew B, Kuruvilla B, *et al.* Chewing tobacco, alcohol, and the risk of erythroplakia. *Cancer Epidemiol Biomarkers Prev* 2000;**9**:639–45.
97. Thomas G, Hashibe M, Jacob BJ, *et al.* Risk factors for multiple oral premalignant lesions. *Int J Cancer* 2003;**107**:285–91.
98. Jacob BJ, Straif K, Thomas G, *et al.* Betel quid without tobacco as a risk factor for oral pre-cancers. *Oral Oncol* 2004;**40**:697–704.
99. Sudbo J, Kildal W, Johannessen AC, *et al.* Gross genomic aberrations in precancers: Clinical implications of a long-term follow-up study in oral erythroplakias. *J Clin Oncol* 2002;**20**: 456–62.
100. Qin GZ, Park JY, Chen SY, *et al.* A high prevalence of p53 mutations in pre-malignant oral erythroplakia. *Int J Cancer* 1999;**80**:345–8.
101. Tilakaratne WM, Klinikowski MF, Saku T, *et al.* Oral submucous fibrosis: Review on aetiology and pathogenesis. *Oral Oncol* 2006;**42**:561–8.
102. Rajendran R, Vijayakumar T, Vasudevan DM. An alternative pathogenetic pathway for oral submucous fibrosis (OSMF). *Med Hypotheses* 1989;**30**:35–7.
103. Aziz SR. Coming to America: Betel nut and oral submucous fibrosis. *J Am Dent Assoc* 2010;**141**:423–8.
104. Maher R, Lee AJ, Warnakulasuriya KA, *et al.* Role of areca nut in the causation of oral submucous fibrosis: A case–control study in Pakistan. *J Oral Pathol Med* 1994;**23**:65–9.
105. Vilcek J, Palombella VJ, Henriksen-DeStefano D, *et al.* Fibroblast growth enhancing activity of tumor necrosis factor and its relationship to other polypeptide growth factors. *J Exp Med* 1986;**163**:632–43.
106. Liu CJ, Lee YJ, Chang KW, *et al.* Polymorphism of the MICA gene and risk for oral submucous fibrosis. *J Oral Pathol Med* 2004;**33**:1–6.

K. Alok Pathak, Rehan Kazi, and Richard W. Nason

Introduction

The importance of an intact mandibular arch for functional and aesthetic reasons can hardly be overemphasized. Invasion of the mandible by intraoral carcinoma often necessitates its surgical removal. Central mandibular defects, in particular, result in severe cosmetic disfigurement and functional impairment [1]. For almost a century before the pioneering work of Marchetta, even uninvolved mandibles were resected routinely as part of a commando operation for their possible involvement by subperiosteal lymphatics [2]. Marchetta proposed that the mandible was invaded by direct extension [2].

Subsequently, McGregor and MacDonald identified the periodontal membrane at the gingival crest on the occlusal surface as the most preferred site of tumour invasion in the non-irradiated mandible [3]. They could not identify any definite route of entry or pattern of invasion in the irradiated mandible [3]. Brown et al. described the point of abutment (junction of the attached and reflected mucosa) as the preferable point of entry [4]. They inferred that tumours of the tongue, floor of mouth and buccal mucosa invade the mandible directly, whereas those of the

K.A. Pathak (✉)
Head and Neck Surgical Oncology, CancerCare Manitoba, Department of Surgery,
University of Manitoba, Winnipeg, MB, Canada
e-mail: alok.pathak@cancercare.mb.ca

R. Kazi
Head and Neck Cancer, Manipal University, Manipal, India
e-mail: drrehankazi@gmail.com

R.W. Nason
Department of Surgery, Faculty of Medicine, University of Manitoba,
ON2042 CancerCare MB 675 McDermot Avenue, Winnipeg, MB, Canada
e-mail: nasonrw@cc.umanitoba.ca

© The Author(s) 2012
K.A. Pathak, R.W. Nason (eds.), *Controversies in Oral Cancer*,
Head and Neck Cancer Clinics, DOI 10.1007/978-81-322-2574-4_3

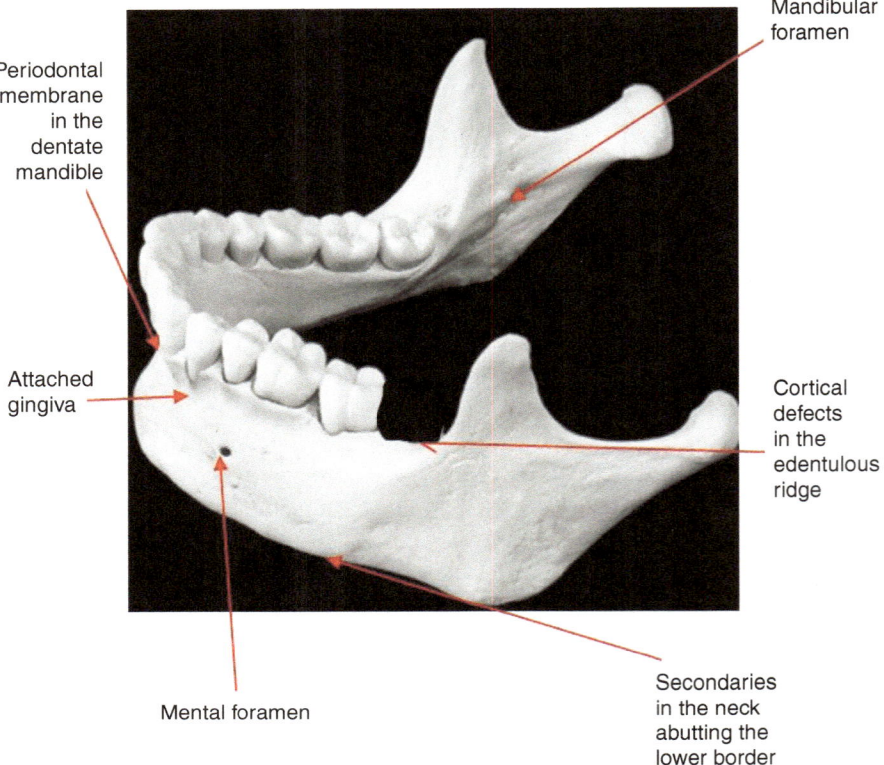

Mandibular foramen

Periodontal membrane in the dentate mandible

Attached gingiva

Cortical defects in the edentulous ridge

Mental foramen

Secondaries in the neck abutting the lower border

Fig. 3.1 Sites of invasion of the mandible

alveolus and retromolar trigone (RMT) invade through the occlusal surface. They found that the presence of teeth did not affect the pattern of tumour invasion and the increased height of the dentate mandible did not delay the invasive pattern of bone involvement [4]. The possible sites of invasion of the mandible by an oral tumour are shown in Fig. 3.1.

The mucoperiosteum overlying the alveolar part of mandible forms the attached gingiva and is reflected inferiorly to form the lining of the cheek (buccal mucosa). This line of reflection runs along the lower buccal–gingival sulcus. Below this level of mucosal reflection the mandible is covered only with periosteum and is supplied by rich anastomoses of endosteal and periosteal vessels. The blood supply to a child's mandible is multifocal in origin. The main endosteal component is supplied by the inferior dental artery, which arises from the first part of the maxillary artery. The maxillary artery forms a rich anastomosis with the second component of the blood supply that arises from the subperiosteal plexus of vessels supplied by the facial, buccal, lingual and mylohyoid arteries [5]. Brookes estimated the arterial supply from the inferior dental artery to be adequate for a 13-year-old child's mandible, but in an adult its contribution to the blood supply is only 4.72 % [6]. Bradley postulated that the inferior dental artery suffers from a marked collagenosis of its

Table 3.1 Factors determining the surgical approach to oral cancers

Access
  Location
  Size
  Mouth opening
  Prominent incisors
  Bony erosion and paramandibular spread
  Dentition and mandibular height
  Invasion of inferior alveolar nerve
  Deep infiltration into extrinsic muscles
  Post-radiation recurrent disease

wall almost 15 years earlier than other branches of the carotid artery, possibly due to abnormal stress factors being exerted within the wall [7]. Thus, from middle age onwards, the blood supply to the mandible is mainly from the subperiosteal plexus of vessels. It is suggested that the main supply to the lower border of the mandible arises from this plexus [6]. Barttelbort and Ariyan found that the lower border of the mandible has 50 % of cross-sectional area and contributes maximally to the strength of the mandible [8].

Management of oral cancer underwent a paradigm shift with these newer insights into the surgical anatomy of the mandible and the routes of mandibular invasion. Factors determining the surgical approach to oral cancer are outlined in Table 3.1. The possibility of adequately removing selected oral cancers without disrupting mandibular continuity and the muscular attachments led to the popularity of mandibular arch-preserving procedures for preventing cosmetic and functional problems resulting from segmental mandibular resection. When comparing segmental mandibulectomy with marginal mandibulectomy, a 12-month follow up shows that even though microvascular reconstruction of the mandible has made the former a less morbid procedure, the latter procedure results in less functional problems and better quality of life by preserving mandibular continuity and muscular attachments [8, 9].

Mandibular preservation offers the following advantages: Preservation of the anatomy; avoidance of complex mandibular reconstruction, which results in decreased operative time, reduced hospital stay and decreased postoperative morbidity; and better long-term aesthetic and functional results. All mandible-preservation procedures require preserved mandible of at least 1 cm height with no clinical/radiological evidence of bone erosion. For mandibulotomy and marginal mandibulectomy, a non-irradiated, dentate mandible with adequate height is ideal. Pipe stem edentulous mandibles are not suitable for marginal mandibulectomy, as the remaining mandible is not strong enough for mastication.

Mandible-Preserving Approaches to Oral Cancer

Preoperative assessment includes bi-digital clinical examination and radiological evaluation by orthopantogram (panorex) and computerized tomography (CT scan), thereby combining the sensitivity of clinical examination with the specificity of CT scan [10, 11]. The final decision to proceed with mandible preservation is taken after an intraoperative bi-digital assessment is done under anaesthesia, based on the ability to achieve 3-dimensional adequate margins of at least 5 mm.

Broadly, these approaches can be divided into two major categories: Peroral and transoral–transcervical approaches.

Per-oral Approach

Access to the oral cavity is limited by the mandible. Adequate mouth opening is essential for proper assessment and resection of oral cancer. For optimal exposure, nasal endotracheal intubation is preferable if a preoperative tracheostomy is not planned. Oral bite blocks provide good exposure, stabilize the jaw and free the surgeon's hands. Another good aid for retraction of the anterior tongue is a silk suture that can be grasped with a haemostat and pulled anteriorly. It is ideal for anteriorly sited, superficial lesions close to the midline, especially soft tissue tumours, including those requiring symphyseal marginal mandibulectomy or anterior maxillary alveolectomy.

Transoral–Transcervical Approach

Lip-Split Approach

For posteriorly placed deep-seated cancers I prefer a lip split to raise the cheek flap for optimal exposure and adequate soft tissue margins. The lip-split technique was first described by Roux who combined the neck incision with a mid-lower lip incision to reflect the entire flap laterally to allow tumour resection and neck dissection [12]. McGregor modified the incision by curving the midline lower lip incision in the labio-mental crease on the side of the planned reflection [13]. Robson attempted a more aesthetic step by moving the incision in the lower lip and chin more laterally to start medial to the ipsilateral lip commissure and descend in the relaxed skin crease to meet the neck incision [14].

Lip-Split Mandibulotomy Approach

The lip-split approach described above can be combined with ipsilateral mandibulotomy. It involves lingual–mandibular release. It is ideal for posteriorly situated tongue lesions not involving the floor of the mouth or for more anterior lesions with limited mouth opening.

An incision is made through the floor of the mouth up to the anterior tonsillar pillar, and the lip–mandible–buccal mucosa complex is swung laterally to access the posterior part of the oral cavity. Stair-step, vertical, and arrowhead mandibulectomy (Fig. 3.2a–c) have been described. Step mandibulectomy often results in loss of one or more teeth because of which the other two techniques are preferred. The mandible can be split in the midline, paramedian or lateral positions. However, in order to preserve the neurovascular bundle of the mandibular inferior alveolar nerve, mandibular cuts are placed anterior to the mental foramen area by at least 7 mm to avoid

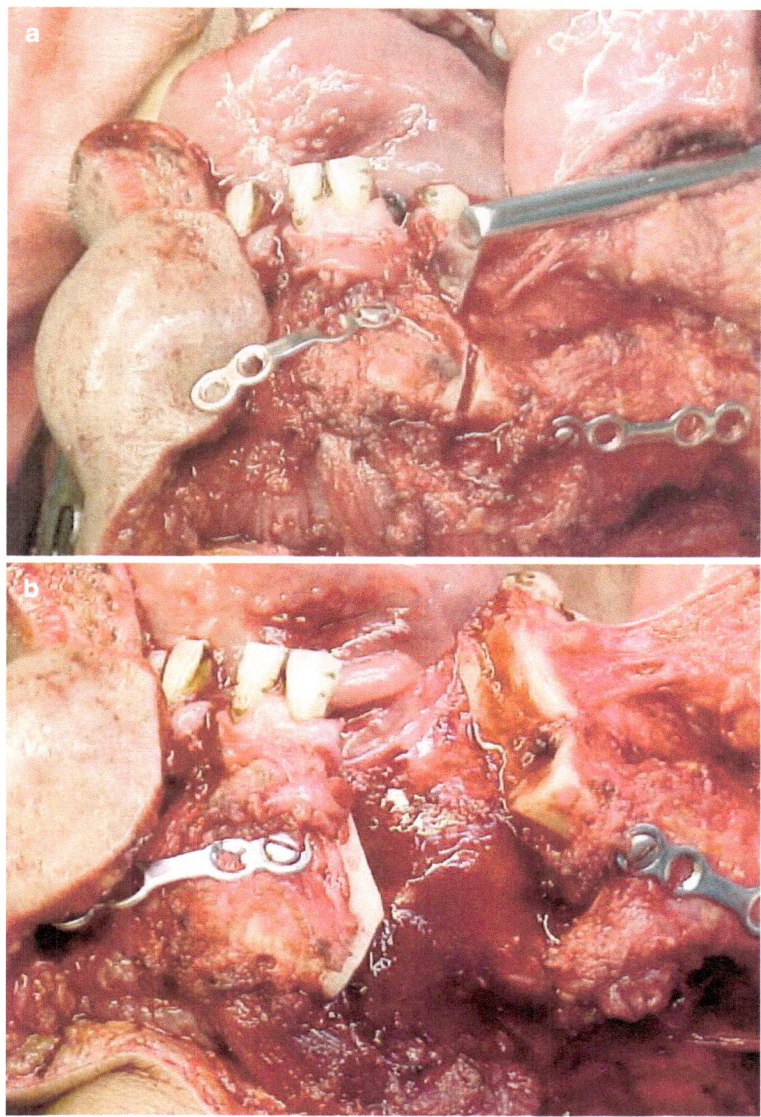

Fig. 3.2 (**a**) Marking for left mandibulotomy. (**b**) Osteotomy completed

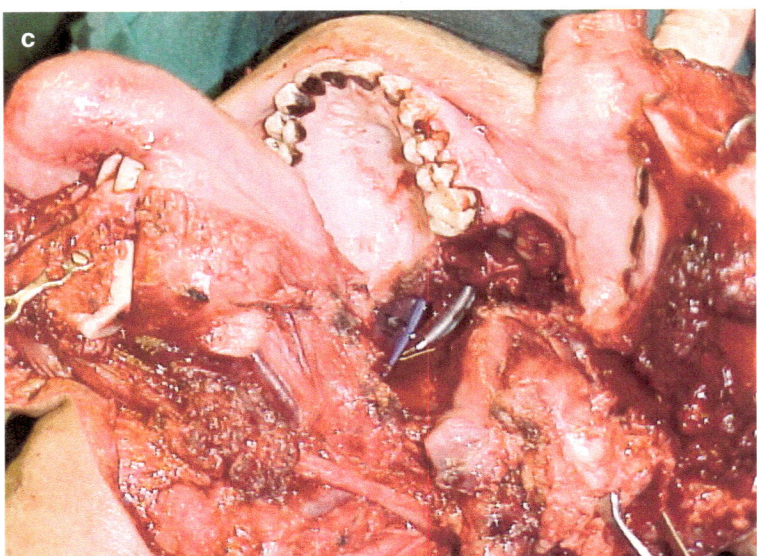

Fig. 3.2 (**c**) Access to the posterior oral cavity

injury to the mental nerve as it curves back to emerge from its bony foramen. The mandibular swing also provides access to the posterior maxilla, pterygoid plates, oropharynx and parapharyngeal space [15]. Median labio-mandibulo-glossotomy was first described by Trotter in 1929 and it is still used to access the posterior oropharynx and anterior cervical spine [16].

Pull-Through Approach

This method was described originally in 1975 by Scheunemann [17] and modified in 1984 by Stanley [18] to allow in-continuity resection of oral cavity tumours with the cervical lymph nodes, while avoiding a lower lip-split incision. A visor flap is developed after a mastoid-to-mastoid neck incision while avoiding the labial and buccal intraoral releasing incisions. It provides good access to the posterior tongue and is suitable for posterior tongue lesions. The tongue and floor of the mouth are released by dividing the mylohoid, genioglossus and geniohyoid muscles. The tongue is then pulled below the mandible into the neck (Fig. 3.3a, b). Care needs to be taken to avoid damage to the lingual arteries and nerves, and the hypoglossal nerves. After excision, the floor of the mouth needs to be repaired/reconstructed meticulously and the tongue needs to be re-suspended to avoid compromised swallowing and speech [18, 19]. In addition to compromised lingual function, dehiscence of the floor of the mouth results in an orocervical fistula, and tongue oedema results in a compromised airway.

Marginal Mandibulectomy

Marginal mandibulectomy is a mandible-preserving procedure for resecting oral cancers that come close to the mandible or involve it superficially. Indications for

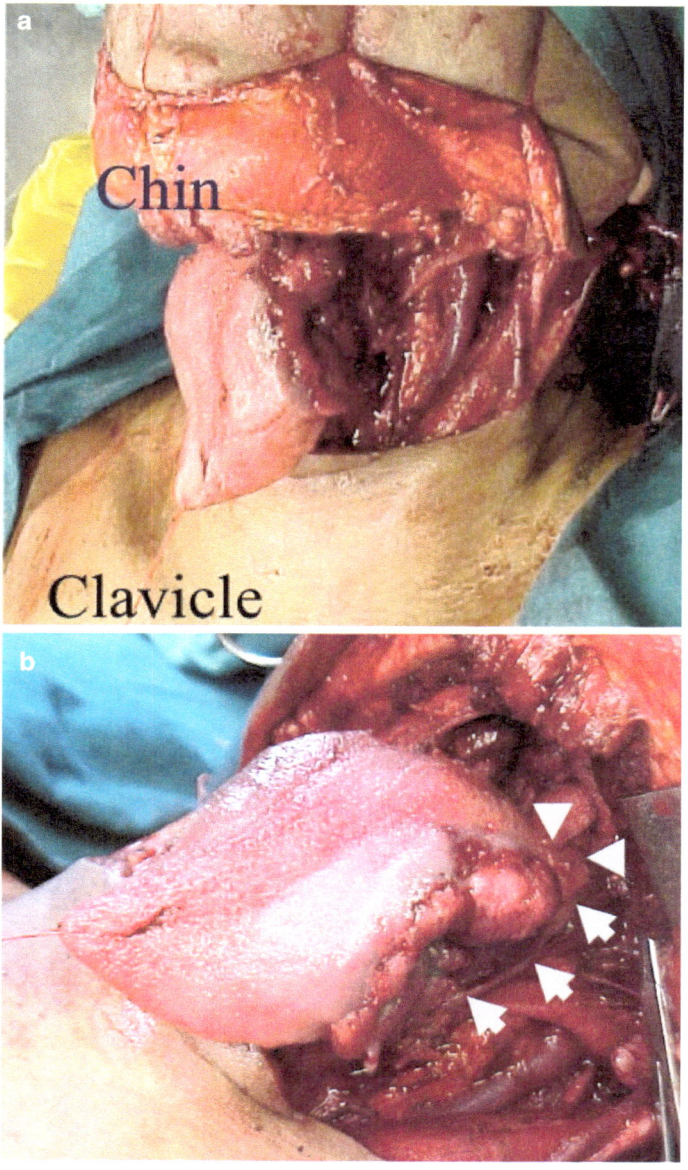

Fig. 3.3 (a) Lingual mandibular release. (b) Close up of posterior tongue cancer

marginal mandibulectomy include superficial alveolar carcinoma, selected carcinoma of the gingival buccal sulcus, carcinoma of the floor of the mouth and carcinoma of the buccal mucosa [20–23]. It is an oncologically sound procedure, which
is more radical than the periosteal stripping described by Brown et al. [24] and less
morbid than segmental mandibulectomy for selected oral cancers.

Various series have reported comparable local control rates in patients with marginal and segmental resections, and oncological safety is not compromised by marginal mandibulectomy [25–30]. Indications for segmental and marginal mandibulectomies have been often debated [31], but in the authors' opinion these procedures are mutually exclusive and are meant for different indications, and it is inappropriate to compare their oncological outcomes. Marginal mandibulectomy is best suited for cancers that are proximal to non-radiated mandibles or that erode the mandible superficially, in which case it is possible to get adequate margins, while preserving adequate mandibular mass and continuity to withstand the strain of mastication. Segmental mandibulectomy with microvascular mandibular reconstruction is indicated when marginal mandibulectomy is either not possible or is oncologically unsafe. Microvascular free-tissue transfer prolongs surgery, results in added donor site morbidity, and puts an additional burden on healthcare resources. For these reasons, feasibility of mandibular reconstruction is not an indication for segmental mandibulectomy.

Marginal mandibulectomy can be classified in the following ways:

- Vertical
  - Lingual plate
  - Buccal plate [32]
- Horizontal
  - Rim resection
  - Lower border-preserving resection
  - Oblique
  - Step

Assessment for the appropriateness and type of marginal mandibulectomy is based on the position of the tumour in the oral cavity, its relationship with the underlying mandible, and mandibular height and contact of the tumour with the mandible. For lesions in proximity with either the lingual or buccal cortex, a lingual or buccal plate excision is adequate. Should the alveolar process be involved, a formal excision of the alveolar process along with the buccal or lingual plate is required. Assessment of paramandibular spread requires good exposure; a cheek flap is often needed for laterally and posteriorly placed lesions or if the mouth opening is limited. Adequate soft tissue and bone margins are essential for oncological safety of the procedure. All attempts should be made to preserve the mandibular canal and mandibular periosteum (Fig. 3.4a, b). We always attempt to preserve at least 10 mm of the inferior border of the mandible, which accounts for ~50 % of the cross-sectional area of the mandible and mandibular strength [7]. The preserved mandible should have adequate strength and blood supply to withstand the forces of mastication. Buccal plate excision leaves the lingual soft tissue attachment and the underlying periosteal plexus intact; and in many cases, the inferior dental artery that runs close to the lingual plate towards the lower border of the mandible is preserved [33]. Proper instruments, such as an oscillating saw or a high-speed drill, are required.

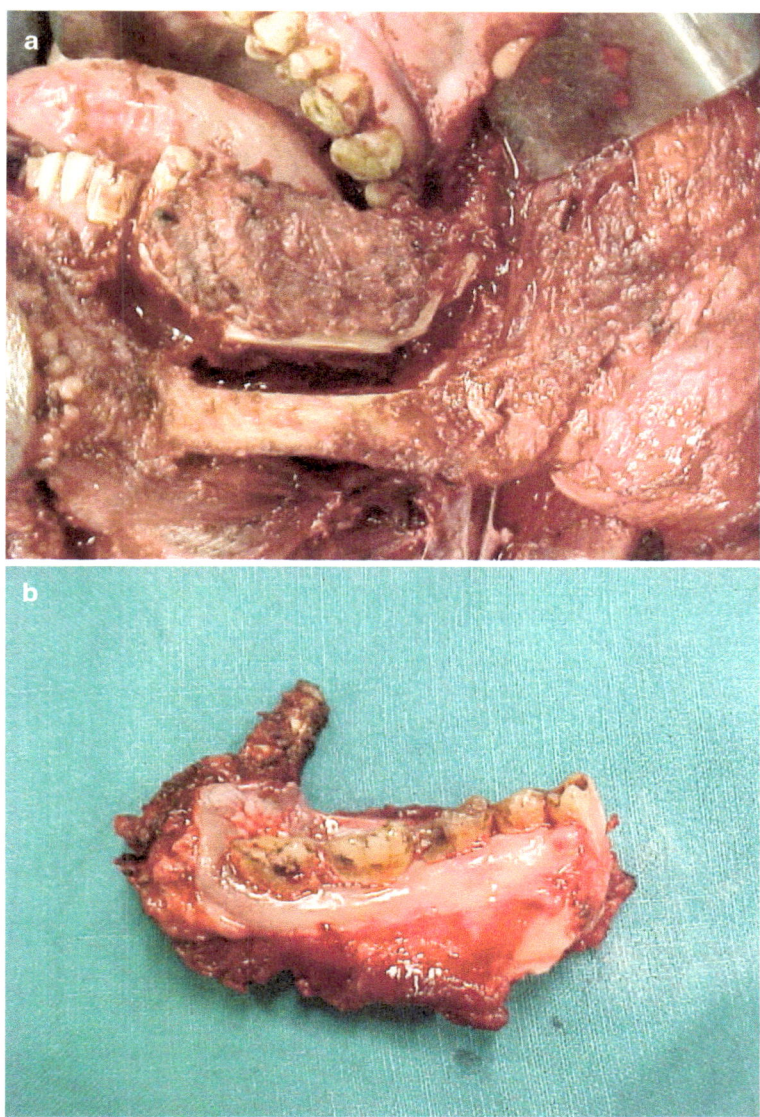

Fig. 3.4 (**a**) Marginal mandibulectomy for buccal cancer. (**b**) Specimen

Appropriate soft cover for the mandible is essential after the procedure to avoid subsequent mandibular exposure and osteomyelitis.

In properly selected cases, marginal mandibulectomy can achieve good disease control without compromising on the aesthetics and function of the mandible. Because it is a shorter procedure, it puts less strain on resources and does not require complex microsurgical reconstruction. It offers excellent 2-year and 5-year cause-specific survival (85.6 % and 72.2 %, respectively) and an overall local control rate of 89.4 %. Our team found the post-marginal mandibulectomy cause-specific survival at 5 years to be significantly better for gingival buccal cancers than for floor of the mouth cancers (76.1 % versus 42.7 %; p = 0.041) [23]. Mandible preservation is an excellent alternative to segmental mandibulectomy in selected early oral cancers.

Contraindications to mandibular preservation include the following:

- Gross involvement of the mandible
- Extensive paramandibular spread involving more than two surfaces of the mandible
- Alveolar process resorption (pipe stem mandible)
- Recent tooth extraction
- Irradiated mandible
- Tumour abutting bone on more than two aspects
- Inability to preserve the inferior alveolar artery.

References

1. Pathak KA, Shah BC, Date AS, *et al.* Primary reconstruction of small mandibular defects by using mandibular remnant. *J Surg Oncol* 2006;**93**:593–5.
2. Marchetta FC, Sako K, Badillo J. Periosteal lymphatics of the mandible and intraoral carcinoma. *Am J Surg* 1964;**108**:505–7.
3. McGregor AD, MacDonald DG. Routes of entry of squamous cell carcinoma to the mandible. *Head Neck Surg* 1988;**10**:294–301.
4. Brown JS, Lowe D, Kalavrezos N, *et al.* Patterns of invasion and routes of tumor entry into the mandible by oral squamous cell carcinoma. *Head Neck* 2002;**24**:370–83.
5. Cohen L. Methods of investigating the vascular architecture of the mandible. *J Dent Res* 1959;**38**:920–31.
6. Brookes M. *The blood supply in bone.* London: Butterworths; 1971.
7. Bradley JC. The clinical significance of age changes in the vascular supply to the mandible. *Int J Oral Surg* 1981;**10** (Suppl 1):71–6.
8. Barttelbort SW, Ariyan S. Mandible preservation with oral cavity carcinoma: Rim mandibulectomy versus sagittal mandibulectomy. *Am J Surg* 1993;**166**:411–15.
9. Namaki S, Matsumoto M, Ohba H, *et al.* Masticatory efficiency before and after surgery in oral cancer patients: Comparative study of glossectomy, marginal mandibulectomy and segmental mandibulectomy. *J Oral Sci* 2004;**46**:113–17.
10. van den Brekel MW, Runne RW, Smeele LE, *et al.* Assessment of tumour invasion into the mandible: The value of different imaging techniques. *Eur Radiol* 1998;**8**:1552.
11. Jones AS, England J, Hamilton J, *et al.* Mandibular invasion in patients with oral and oropharyngeal squamous carcinoma. *Clin Otolaryngol Allied Sci* 1997;**22**:239.
12. Roux PJ. Cited in Butlin HT, Spencer GJ (eds). *Diseases of the tongue.* London: Cassell; 1900:359.
13. McGregor IA, MacDonald DG. Mandibular osteotomy in the surgical approach to the oral cavity. *Head Neck Surg* 1983;**5**:457–62.
14. Robson MC. An easy access incision for the removal of some intraoral malignant tumors. *Plast Reconstr Surg* 1979;**64**:834–5.
15. Dingman DL, Conley J. Lateral approach to the pterygomaxillary region. *Ann Otol Rhinol Laryngol* 1970;**79**:967–9.

16. Trotter W. Operations for malignant diseases of the pharynx. *Br J Surg* 1929;**16**:485–95.
17. Scheunemann H. Pull-through surgery in mouth floor-tongue neoplasms. *Acta Stomatol Belg* 1975;**72**:229–30.
18. Stanley RB. Mandibular lingual releasing approach to oral and oropharyngeal carcinomas. *Laryngoscope* 1984;**94**:596–600.
19. Devine JC, Rogers SN, McNally D, *et al*. A comparison of aesthetic, functional and patient subjective outcomes following lip-splitting mandibulotomy and mandibular lingual releasing access procedures. *Int J Oral Maxillofac Surg* 2001;**30**:199–204.
20. Shaha AR. Marginal mandibulectomy for carcinoma of the floor of the mouth. *J Surg Oncol* 1992;**49**:116–19.
21. Pathak KA, Agarwal R, Deshpande MS. Marginal mandibulectomy for lateral sulcus tumors. *Eur J Surg Oncol* 2004;**30**:804–6.
22. Bahadur S. Marginal resection of the mandible in oral cancer. *Indian J Cancer* 1994;**31**:235–9.
23. Pathak KA, Shah BC. Marginal mandibulectomy: 11 years of institutional experience. *J Oral Maxillofac Surg* 2009;**67**:962–7.
24. Brown JS, Griffith JF, Phelps PD, *et al*. A comparison of different imaging modalities and direct inspection after periosteal stripping in predicting the invasion of the mandible by oral squamous cell carcinoma. *Br J Oral Maxillofac Surg* 1994;**32**:347–59.
25. O'Brien CJ, Adams JR, McNeil EB, *et al*. Influence of bone invasion and extent of mandibular resection on local control of cancers of the oral cavity and oropharynx. *Int J Oral Maxillofac Surg* 2003;**32**:492–7.
26. Dubner S, Heller KS. Local control of squamous cell carcinoma following marginal and segmental mandibulectomy. *Head Neck* 1993;**15**:29–32.
27. Ord RA, Sarmadi M, Papadimitrou J. A comparison of segmental and marginal bony resection for oral squamous cell carcinoma involving the mandible. *J Oral Maxillofac Surg* 1997;**55**:470–7.
28. Shingaki S, Nomura T, Takada M, *et al*. Squamous cell carcinomas of the mandibular alveolus: Analysis of prognostic factors. *Oncology* 2002;**62**:17–24.
29. Wolff D, Hassfeld S, Hofele C. Influence of marginal and segmental mandibular resection on the survival rate in patients with squamous cell carcinoma of the inferior parts of the oral cavity. *J Craniomaxillofac Surg* 2004;**32**:318–23.
30. Muñoz Guerra MF, Naval Gías L, Campo FR, *et al*. Marginal and segmental mandibulectomy in patients with oral cancer: A statistical analysis of 106 cases. *J Oral Maxillofac Surg* 2003;**61**:1289–96.
31. Wax MK, Bascom DA, Myers LL. Marginal mandibulectomy vs segmental mandibulectomy: Indications and controversies. *Arch Otolaryngol Head Neck Surg* 2002:**128**:600–3.
32. Pathak KA, Deshpande MS, Mathur N, *et al*. Buccal plate excision for buccal paramandibular spread. *J Surg Oncol* 2006;**94**:257–9.
33. Gowgiel JM. The position and course of the mandibular canal. *J Oral Implantol* 1992;**18**:383–5.

Surgical Management of Oral Cancer

4

Richard W. Nason and K. Alok Pathak

Introduction

Oral cancer represents a heterogeneous and complex group of tumours, variable in their behaviour and potentially lethal. In a historical cohort of 700 patients from the population-based cancer registry of the province of Manitoba, the 5-year disease-specific survival was 63 %. Survival was 74 % for stage I, 59 % for stage II, 52 % for stage III and 29 % for stage IV disease (p=0.0000). A number of factors interacted to determine the outcome in this patient population. Major prognostic factors, as determined by multivariate analysis, included (i) gender, (ii) age, (iii) site in the oral cavity, (iv) clinical stage, and (v) initial treatment modality. Results were consistently superior with surgery. Radiotherapy as a single treatment modality was associated with an adverse outcome (HR 2.0; 95 % CI 1.8–2.7; p=0.000). In 311 patients treated with surgery alone and 148 patients treated with surgery and adjunctive radiotherapy, involved surgical margins had a significant impact on survival after controlling for age and stage of disease (HR 2.0; 95 % CI 1.3–3.0; p=0.0022) [1, 2].

The treatment plan for any patient with oral cancer involves treatment of the primary and of the neck. Treatment of the neck is discussed in detail in other volumes of this series. Resection of oral cancer should generally not be undertaken unless a negative or clear margin around the tumour can be obtained. Unlike the other prognostic factors described above, the status of the margin is, in part, under

R.W. Nason
Department of Surgery, Faculty of Medicine, University of Manitoba,
ON2042 CancerCare MB, 675 McDermot Avenue, Winnipeg, MB, Canada
e-mail: nasonrw@cc.umanitoba.ca

K.A. Pathak (✉)
Head and Neck Surgical Oncology, CancerCare Manitoba, Department of Surgery,
University of Manitoba, Winnipeg, MB, Canada
e-mail: alok.pathak@cancercare.mb.ca

© The Author(s) 2012
K.A. Pathak, R.W. Nason (eds.), *Controversies in Oral Cancer*,
Head and Neck Cancer Clinics, DOI 10.1007/978-81-322-2574-4_4

direct control of the surgeon. There is no single definition of an adequate resection margin. As defined by Yuen, the optimal resection margin should not compromise local control from an adequate resection or cause unnecessary functional morbidity from too much resection [3].

Defining the Adequate Surgical Resection Margin

Microscopic tumour at or close to the resection margin increases the chance of local recurrence by a factor of two or more in most series [4–13]. The impact of margin status on survival lacks a common consensus. A decrease in survival was noted in our historical cohort of oral cancer patients in Manitoba. A decrease in survival with positive margins has also been reported by others [5–7, 14, 15], but not by all investigators [9, 12, 16–18]. A close, but clear margin, is also felt to contribute to an adverse outcome. This fact has to be considered in establishing the adequate depth and width of surgical resection. The most widely accepted definition of a close margin is a tumour within 5 mm of the resection margin [4–7, 11, 19, 20]. Admittedly, this is an arbitrary designation, and when recurrence rates are sited specifically for close margins, they are generally less than the rate observed for patients with a tumour at the inked resection margin [3–5, 18]. This is important, as patients with close surgical margins are generally considered as candidates for adjunctive radiotherapy.

Our team examined the impact of the width of the surgical margin on outcome in our historical cohort of oral cancer patients from Manitoba [2]. A step-by-step increase in survival was demonstrated with each additional millimetre of clear surgical margin. After controlling for other confounding factors, each 1 mm increase in the clear surgical margin decreased the risk of death at 5 years by 8 % (HR 0.92; 95 % CI 0.86–0.99; p=0.021) [2]. Using a Cox proportional hazard model in this study, three groups were identified with similar survival probabilities: the clear margin was defined as >4 mm and was associated with the best survival probability; patients with positive margins had a 2.5-fold increase in risk of death; and patients with margins ≤3 mm had a 1.5-fold increase in risk of death. This study challenged the more traditional definition of a close margin as <5 mm, as proposed by Looser and Loree [4, 5]. This is an important consideration as radiation is often considered for an inadequate or close margin. Several reports have suggested that recurrence rates are reduced with the addition of radiation in the presence of an inadequate margin [21–23]. In our series of oral cancer patients in Manitoba, adjunctive radiation for microscopically positive or close margins did not impact survival or disease control. A similar conclusion was reached by Brown and co-workers from Liverpool, who documented an adverse impact on outcome in their intermediate risk patients [24].

From a practical point of view, resection of an oral cancer needs to include at least a 1 cm and preferably a wider 1.5 cm margin of grossly normal tissue. It is important to remember that the clinical margin necessary to achieve an adequate histological margin on permanent pathology needs to consider the fact that the surgical margin shrinks to the order of 40–50 % when placed in formalin [20]. Recurrences at the primary site most frequently involve the deep resection margin [11, 25]. A 3-dimensional resection is essential. Important tumour- and patient-related factors that are consistently associated with positive margins need to be considered when planning a surgical resection. These include the following: (i) The status of the tumour–host interface; (ii) tumour volume; (iii) proximity to the mandible; and (iv) a posterior location in the oral cavity. These factors, in conjunction with the patient's expectation of a functional outcome, will influence a surgical approach with a goal of achieving a negative margin.

Frozen section assessment of margins intra-operatively is used to facilitate the exercise of achieving a negative margin. In our own outcome data [26], intra-operative use of frozen section did not influence margin status on permanent section or outcome. The reason for this is that a frozen section tends to emphasize the mucosal and not the deep resection margin. In addition, the common practice of assessing the patient's resection margin does not identify the patient with a close margin. Our current practices need to be re-examined to emphasize involvement and proximity to the deep resection margin.

Principles of Surgical Management

The surgical management of oral cancer involves the following four interrelated and often overlapping steps: (i) Exposure, (ii) exploration, (iii) resection, and (iv) reconstruction.

Exploration starts well before the operative procedure with clinical staging. A complete history and physical examination with thorough evaluation of the upper aero-digestive tract is necessary to evaluate the extent of the primary tumour as well as exclude the presence of second primary malignancies. Imaging of the neck is essential. CT, MRI and ultrasound, as reviewed in detail by van den Brekel and co-workers, are all superior to physical examination in assessing the status of the cervical lymph nodes [27]. A panorex of the mandible is obtained if the tumour approaches or clinically involves the mandible. The status, and mainly height of the mandible, in this predominantly edentulous population, has important surgical implications. It is emphasized that this investigation is not useful in detecting early stages of mandibular involvement. It is the opinion of our group that early and sub-clinical involvement of the mandible does not influence treatment decisions and outcome [28, 29].

Exploration also involves a thorough understanding and review of the pathology. Tumours >2–4 mm in thickness are associated with a higher incidence of occult cervical metastases [30, 31]. The status of the tumour–host interface has important therapeutic and prognostic implications [32, 33]. A tumour with a broad pushing margin will have a lower probability of occult cervical metastases than one with a border invading in sheets and cords into the adjacent stroma. In addition, it would be easier to obtain a clear surgical margin in the presence of a broad pushing margin.

The mandible is a key structure in the pathology of oral cancer and its surgical management. Maintenance of continuity is central to a good functional and cosmetic outcome. The mandible is the skeletal foundation for facial contour in the lower third of the face and provides the attachments through which the tongue muscles function. Management of the mandible in oral cancer is addressed in more detail in another chapter of this series. Briefly, in squamous cell carcinoma of the floor of the mouth, the lower alveolus, retromolar trigone and buccal sulcus tumours will be directly applied to bone. In the presence of clinical or radiological evidence of gross mandibular invasion, resection of the mandible is indicated. In addition, it is often necessary to consider resection of the mandible to achieve an adequate resection margin. From a practical point of view, this is a consideration for a tumour within 1–1.5 cm of the mandible. For this purpose, marginal resection is a sound oncological procedure, assuming the mandibular height is adequate and an adequate soft tissue margin can be achieved. Biomechanical studies suggest that the strength of the remaining mandible is not compromised if the height remaining is at least 10 mm. This procedure is safe in the presence of early or minimal bone involvement [28, 29]. Full-thickness resection of bone or segmental mandibulectomy is indicated if the vertical height of the mandible is inadequate, or in cases where gross clinical and radiological involvement of bone is present. Segmental mandibulectomy is also indicated in the presence of treatment failure after radiotherapy.

There are several surgical approaches to the oral cavity. The approach is selected on the basis of the ability to resect the tumour with an adequate surgical margin. Small anterior lesions can be resected through the natural incision of the mouth—the per-oral approach. Larger lesions require wider exposure for adequate excision. A midline lip-splitting incision with elevation of a cheek flap can provide wide exposure. Additional exposures bring the management of the mandible back into consideration. The floor of the mouth can be dropped or pulled through into the neck. For this procedure to be used safely, an adequate margin of normal tissue of >1–1.5 cm between the inner aspect of the mandible and the tumour must be present. An anterior mandibulotomy with a mandibular swing provides wide exposure for more posteriorly located lesions. The key to the use of this procedure is again an adequate margin of normal tissue between the lingual aspect of the mandible and the edge of the tumour.

After an adequate resection, the final consideration is reconstruction. This too is discussed at length in another section of this monograph. The optimal functional outcome in oral cancer is dependent on how freely mobile the tongue remains and how effectively the mandibular arch is maintained or restored. To achieve this goal, it is extremely important to approach each case of oral cancer with a full complement of reconstructive techniques. These will range from primary closure and transposition of local tissue to pedicled and free flaps. The resection should never be limited or extended to accommodate any single method of reconstruction.

References

1. Binahmed A, Nason R, Abdoh A. The clinical significance of the positive surgical margin in oral cancer. *Oral Oncology* 2006;**43**:780–4.
2. Nason R, Binahmed A, Abdoh A. What is the adequate margin of surgical resection in oral cancer. *Oral Surg Oral Med Oral Pathol Oral Radiol Endod* 2009;**105**:625–9.
3. Yuen PW, Lam KY, Chan ACL, *et al.* Clinicopathological analysis of local spread of carcinoma of the tongue. *Am J Surg* 1998;**175**:242–4.
4. Looser KG, Shah JP, Strong EW. The significance of "positive" margins in surgically resected epidermoid carcinomas. *Head Neck* 1978;**1**:107–11.
5. Loree TR, Strong EW. Significance of positive margins in oral cavity squamous carcinoma. *Am J Surg* 1990;**160**:410–14.
6. Chen TY, Emrich LJ, Driscoll DL. The clinical significance of pathological findings in surgically resected margins of the primary tumor in head and neck carcinoma. *Int J Radiation Oncology Biol Phys* 1987;**13**:833–7.
7. Sutton DN, Brown JS, Rogers SN, *et al.* The prognostic implications of the surgical margin in oral squamous cell carcinoma. *Int J Oral Maxillofac Surg* 2003;**32**:30–4.
8. Jones AS. Prognosis in mouth cancer: Tumour factors. *Oral Oncol Eur J Cancer* 1994;**30B**:8115.
9. Yuen APW, Lam KY, Wei WI, *et al.* A comparison of the prognostic significance of tumor diameter, length, width, thickness, area, volume, and clinicopathological features of oral tongue carcinoma. *Am J Surg* 2000;**180**:139–43.
10. Jacobs JR, Ahmad K, Casiano R, *et al.* Implications of positive surgical margins. *Laryngoscope* 1993;**103**:64–8.
11. Ravasz LA, Slootweg PJ, Hordijk GJ, *et al.* The status of the resection margin as a prognostic factor in the treatment of head and neck carcinoma. *J Cranio Max Fac Surg* 1991;**19**:314–18.
12. Spiro RH, Guillamondegui O Jr, Paulino AF, *et al.* Pattern of invasion and margin assessment in patients with oral tongue cancer. *Head Neck* 1999;**21**:408–13.
13. Slootweg PJ, Hordijk GJ, Schade, van Es RJJ, *et al.* Treatment failure and margin status in head and neck cancer. A critical view on the potential value of molecular pathology. *Oral Oncology* 2002;**38**:500–3.
14. Woolgar JA, Brown JS, Scott J, *et al.* Survival, metastasis and recurrence of oral cancer in relation to pathological features. *Ann R Coll Surg Engl* 1995;**77**:325–31.
15. Chandu A, Adams G, Smith ACH. Factors affecting survival in patients with oral cancer: An Australian perspective. *Int J Oral Maxillofac Surg* 2005;**34**:514–20.
16. Jones AS, Bin Hanafi, Z, Nadapalan V, *et al.* Do positive resection margins after ablative surgery for head and neck cancer adversely affect prognosis? A study of 352 patients with recurrent carcinoma following radiotherapy treated by salvage surgery. *Br J Cancer* 1996;**74**: 128–32.
17. Kademani D, Bell RB, Bagberi S, *et al.* Prognostic factors in intraoral squamous cell carcinoma: The influence of histologic grade. *Int J Oral Maxiollofac Surg* 2005;**63**:1599–1605.
18. McMahon J, O'Brien CJ, Pathak I, *et al.* Influence of condition of surgical margins on local recurrence and disease-specific survival in oral and oropharyngeal cancer. *Br J Oral Maxillofac Surg* 2003;**41**:224–31.
19. Meier JD, Oliver DA, Varvares MA. Surgical margin determination in head and neck oncology: Current clinical practice. The results of an international American head and neck society member survey. *Head Neck* 2005;**27**:952–8.
20. Batsakis JG. Surgical excision margins: A pathologist's perspective. *Adv Anat Pathol* 1999;**6**:140–8.
21. Sadeghi A, Kuisk H, Tran LM, *et al.* The role of radiation therapy in squamous cell carcinoma of the upper aero-digestive tract with positive surgical margins. *Am J Clin Oncol (CCT)* 1986;**9**:500–3.

22. Zelefsky MJ, Harrison LB, Fass DE, *et al.* Postoperative radiation therapy for squamous cell carcinomas of the oral cavity and oropharynx: Impact of therapy on patients with positive surgical margins. *Int J Radiation Oncology Biol Phys* 1992;**25**:17–21.
23. Hinerman RW, Mendenhall WM, Morris CG, *et al.* Postoperative irradiation for squamous cell carcinoma of the oral cavity: 35-year experience. *Head Neck* 2004;**26**:984–94.
24. Brown JS, Blackburn TK, Woolgar JA, *et al.* A comparison of outcomes for patients with oral squamous cell carcinoma at intermediate risk of recurrence treated by surgery alone or with post-operative radiotherapy. *Oral Oncology* 2007;**43**:764–73.
25. Woolgar JA, Triantafyllou A. A histopathological appraisal of surgical margins in oral and oropharyngeal cancer resection specimens. *Oral Oncology* 2005;**41**:1034–43.
26. Pathak KA, Nason RW, Penner C, *et al.* Impact of use of frozen section assessment of operative margins on survival in oral cancer. *Oral Surg Oral Med Oral Pathol Oral Radiol Endod* 2009;**107**:235–9.
27. van den Brekel MW, Catelijns JA, Snow GB. Imaging of cervical lymphadenopathy. *Neuroimaging Clin N Am* 1996;**6**:417–34.
28. Ash CS, Nason RW, Abdoh AA, *et al.* Prognostic implications of mandibular invasion in oral cancer. *Head Neck* 2000;**22**:794–8.
29. Pathak KA, Shah BC. Marginal mandibulectomy: 11 years of institutional experience. *J Oral Maxillofac Surg* 2009;**67**:962–7.
30. Byers RM, El-Naggar AK, Lee YY, *et al.* Can we detect or predict the presence of occult nodal metastases in patients with squamous carcinoma of the oral tongue? *Head Neck* 1998;**20**:138–44.
31. O'Brien CJ, Lauer CS, Fredricks S, *et al.* Tumor thickness influences prognosis of T1 and T2 oral cavity cancer—but what thickness? *Head Neck* 2003;**25**:937–45.
32. Bryne M. Is the invasive front of an oral carcinoma the most important area for prognostication? *Oral Dis* 1998;**4**:70–7.
33. Nason RW, Castillo NB, Sako K, *et al.* Cervical node metastases in early squamous cell carcinoma of the floor of the mouth: Predictive value of multiple histopathological parameters. *World J Surg* 1990;**14**:606–9.

Richard W. Nason and K. Alok Pathak

Introduction

The status of the regional lymph nodes is considered to be one of the major prognostic factors of oral cancer. Cure rates drop by ~50 % when the regional lymph nodes are involved. The N0 neck, by definition, means that involvement of the cervical lymph nodes is not evident on clinical assessment, including physical examination and imaging studies. Occult metastases are generally identified at the time of pathological examination of the neck dissection specimen. The long-standing debate concerning the management of the clinically negative neck centres on two basic and interrelated themes. The first is not a necessity in the timing of lymphadenectomy—the question of elective treatment of the neck versus a 'wait and watch' approach. The second is the anatomical extent of treatment, if occult metastatic disease is elected to be treated.

The incidence of occult metastatic disease has been correlated with the size of the primary or T-stage. For larger tumours or deeply invasive tumours, T3 and T4 lesions, the incidence of occult metastases is $\geq$50 %. In smaller tumours (<4 cm), T1 and T2 lesions, the incidence of occult metastases is in the order of 30 % as determined by standard pathological assessment of lymphadenectomy specimens [1–3]. The incidence of treatment failure with observation of the N0 neck may even be higher, in the order of 44–50 % [4–6].

R.W. Nason
Department of Surgery, Faculty of Medicine, University of Manitoba,
ON2042 CancerCare MB, 675 McDermot Avenue, Winnipeg, MB, Canada
e-mail: nasonrw@cc.umanitoba.ca

K.A. Pathak (✉)
Head and Neck Surgical Oncology, CancerCare Manitoba, Department of Surgery,
University of Manitoba, Winnipeg, MB, Canada
e-mail: alok.pathak@cancercare.mb.ca

© The Author(s) 2012   51
K.A. Pathak, R.W. Nason (eds.), *Controversies in Oral Cancer*,
Head and Neck Cancer Clinics, DOI 10.1007/978-81-322-2574-4_5

The Biological Significance of Occult Metastases

Poor prognostic factors, such as extracapsular spread, may be present in the absence of clinically evident disease. Gourin et al. described extracapsular spread in 43 % of 337 patients undergoing elective neck dissection [7]. Disease-free survival for patients in this series with occult metastatic disease was 36 % versus 62 % for patients staged N0 (p<0.0001). Woolgar described extracapsular spread in 34 % of patients with metastatic lymph nodes ≤10 mm in size [8]. A similar impact in overall survival was demonstrated by microscopic evidence of extracapsular spread when compared with patients with macroscopic evidence of extracapsular disease. The extent of neck disease may be greater at the time of neck failure if observation is elected. Andersen, while evaluating 47 patients with regional failure in the neck after observation, noted adverse prognostic factors in 77 %, which included extracapsular spread in 49 % [9]. Evidence has shown that there may be an increased risk of distant metastases with expectant management of occult metastatic disease [10, 11].

Predicting Occult Metastases

Squamous cell carcinoma (SCC) of the oral cavity is a heterogeneous disease with significant biological variability among patients with similar appearing cancers. Elective treatment of the neck is controversial because of the inability to accurately predict the presence of metastatic disease in the lymph nodes prior to treatment. Physical examination, and to some extent imaging, is dependent on enlargement of the lymph nodes involved with metastases for detection. Imaging criteria for involved lymph nodes include a size of >1/1.5 cm, multiplicity with aggregates of ≥3 lymph nodes, and architectural alterations, including a spherical shape or cystic degeneration. Occult metastases tend to be small, several mm in size, and microscopic deposits of tumour might not lead to architectural change. It is estimated that 50 % of occult metastases are <5 mm in diameter and that 85 % of all metastatic submandibular lymph nodes are <1 cm in diameter [1]. Physical examination is inaccurate, missing lymph node metastases in 50–60 % of patients. Imaging (including CT, MRI and ultrasound) does not detect 20–30 % of metastases [12]. Attention has been directed to assessment of the primary tumour as a means of predicting occult metastases. Tumour thickness, characteristics of the tumour–host interface, and scoring systems incorporating multiple histological parameters have all shown promise in predicting the presence of occult metastases [2, 13–15]. Neck metastases are a consequence of genetic and epigenetic alterations at the cellular level. The use of molecular techniques to describe tumour-specific characteristics, such as metastatic potential, is highly desirable. This science is in its infancy. The study of DNA microwaves and genomic hybridization show promise in this area [16].

In summary, all tumours arising in the oral cavity, irrespective of site, have the potential to metastasize to the regional lymph nodes. Using combinations of clinical, imaging, histopathological and molecular studies, 70–75 % of occult metastases can be predicted at best. In other words, 25–30 % of occult metastases will not be diagnosed. The only currently available method to reliably diagnose occult metastatic disease is histological examination of all lymph nodes dissected by a pathologist in a neck dissection specimen.

Evidence Supporting Elective Neck Dissection

Three commonly cited prospective trials have evaluated elective neck dissection and early oral cancer [5, 6, 17]. They have all failed to show a statistically significant survival advantage. In the Vandenbrouck et al. [5] and Fakih et al. [6] studies, improved outcomes for thick, >4 mm tumours was suggested. It is generally accepted that these series were probably too small, with limitations on follow up to demonstrate a survival benefit. The survival advantage was offset by failure at the primary site, death from second primaries and intercurrent disease. However, these three studies did demonstrate a significant impact on regional control. The incidence of occult metastases in the elective neck dissection group in the three studies was 49 % [5], 33 % [6] and 21 % [17]. Numerous retrospective observational studies have found improved outcomes with elective treatment of the neck [4, 18–22]. In general, they report disease-free survival and the majority of these studies are site-specific to the oral tongue. Two of the more recent studies use multivariate techniques to assess the independent effect of elective neck dissection on survival [21, 22].

There is a bias towards treating the clinically negative neck at present. This is based on the fact that occult metastases do have prognostic significance. The identification of adverse prognostic features, such as extracapsular spread, may justify adjunctive treatment. Salvage treatment of failure is relatively low-ranging, from 20 to 30 % [5, 6, 23, 24]. In addition, evidence supports the fact that treatment of occult metastases improves regional control and probably has a positive impact on overall survival [18–20].

Elective Neck Dissection

Since the description of radical neck dissection in the early 1900s, treatment of the neck has become less radical. Sparing of non-lymphatic and functional structures, the modified radical dissection as initially described by Suarez [25] and subsequently popularized by Bocca et al. [26], characterized the evolution of neck dissections through the 1960s to the 1980s. The past 20 years have seen the evolution of selective neck dissections, procedures which, unlike the first two [25, 26], were designed specifically to address the N0 neck.

The selective neck dissection concept came from Ballantyne and others at MD Anderson and was popularized by Byers and Medina [27]. The selectivity was based on historical observations that metastases from oral cancer follow a predictable pattern. Lindberg's classic study in 1972 demonstrated metastases from oral cancer to the submental and submandibular triangle, and to the upper and mid-jugular chain [28]. Lindberg also described the presence of 'skip metastases', in which metastatic tumour could skip the upper echelon of lymph nodes and be found in the mid-jugular chain [28]. These skip metastases were not found in the lower jugular chain (level IV) or in the posterior triangle of the neck (level V) [29]. In a series of 1119 radical neck dissections for oral SCC, Shah found that level V was not involved when levels I and IV were negative [3]. These studies were the basis for the supraomohyoid neck dissection, or dissection of levels I, II and III, for the management of oral cancer.

In the two decades following the introduction of selective neck dissections, outcome data have shown that the supraomohyoid neck dissection, used for the elective treatment of neck and oral cancer, is as effective as modified neck dissection [1, 30–33]. Most studies report on local recurrence. In patients with pathologically negative nodes or limited disease without extracapsular spread, recurrence rates ranged from 3.2 to 7 %. A generally acceptable rate for recurrence after elective treatment to the neck is ≤5 % [34]. Leemans and Snow compared selective neck dissection with modified radical neck dissection in a meta-analysis of 1179 patients [35]. They concluded that recurrence rates were higher after selective neck dissection. A prospective trial on elective modified neck dissection versus supraomohyoid neck dissection for the management of oral cancer was conducted by the Brazilian Head and Neck Cancer Study Group 1998 [36]. Survival was found to be similar in both the groups. Complications, however, were significantly higher with the more extensive surgery.

Most recurrences after selective neck dissection occur within or adjacent to the field of dissection. Spiro et al. [33, 37] and Byers et al. [38] brought attention to 'risk zones' that might not be addressed with the application of supraomohyoid neck dissection as initially described. Byers showed isolated involvement of level IV or III without involvement of levels I and II. He attributed this to 'skip metastases', whereby lymph nodes, not in the orderly progression of disease, are involved with cancer. Byers and Spiro noted that the nodes behind the jugular vein and anterior to the cervical roots, which they referred to as levels IIB and IIIB, may harbour disease [37, 38]. These investigators highlighted the fact that the classically defined limits, as applied to the supraomohyoid neck dissection, may be inaccurate when applied to certain primary sites, such as the tongue. They proposed an expanded or extended supraomohyoid neck dissection for carcinoma of the oral tongue to include levels I, II, IIB, III, IIIB and IV.

Currently, selective neck dissections are the standard of care for elective treatment of the neck. They appear to be oncologically safe and decrease the morbidity of surgery. The 'selectivity' continues to be defined to standardize the operation, permit flexibility by site, limit recurrence and preserve function. The third and latest consensus on the classification and terminology of neck dissections from the American Head and Neck Society focused on the way in which various selective neck dissections are described [39]. The emphasis is to depict specifically the levels dissected to heighten awareness of the nuances of patterns of lymph node metastases on the basis of site of disease origin.

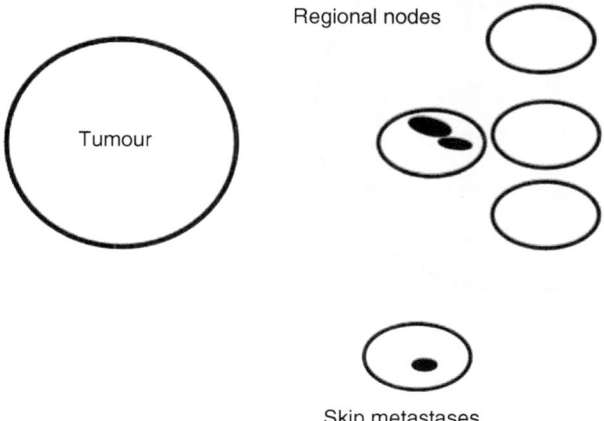

Fig. 5.1 Selective neck dissection is based on the theoretical distribution of cervical node metastases from a specific primary site. This distribution of lymph nodes is represented by the shaded area. Skip metastases outside of the predicted distribution of disease are recognized as a cause of treatment failure

In summary, selective neck dissection, based on the theoretical distribution of the cervical lymph nodes (Fig. 5.1), is the current standard of practice for elective treatment of the neck. This practice presents upwards of 30 lymph nodes to the pathologist for examination for each neck dissected. The accepted incidence of treatment failure after elective treatment of the neck is ~5 %. Skip metastases outside of the predicted distribution of disease are recognized as a cause of treatment failure.

Sentinel Lymph Node Biopsy

Lymphatic mapping and completion lymphadenectomy in the presence of positive sentinel lymph nodes is an attractive alternative to routine elective neck dissection. This concept accepts the orderly progression of metastases from the primary site of the regional draining lymph nodes. Sentinel node biopsy, in contrast to elective neck dissection, is based on the actual and not the theoretical pattern or distribution of lymphatic spread from the individual tumour (Fig. 5.2). This concept recognizes diverse and variable patterns of lymphatic drainage as multiple draining lymphatic pathways and parallel arrays as opposed to 'skip metastases'. Regardless of how non-standard or unique the pattern of lymphatic drainage may be, the sentinel node will always be the site of metastases. In contrast to an elective neck dissection, one or two lymph nodes, representing a small amount of highly predictive tissue, are presented to the pathologist. This facilitates detailed pathological examination of the material submitted, including serial step sectioning, immunocytochemistry and

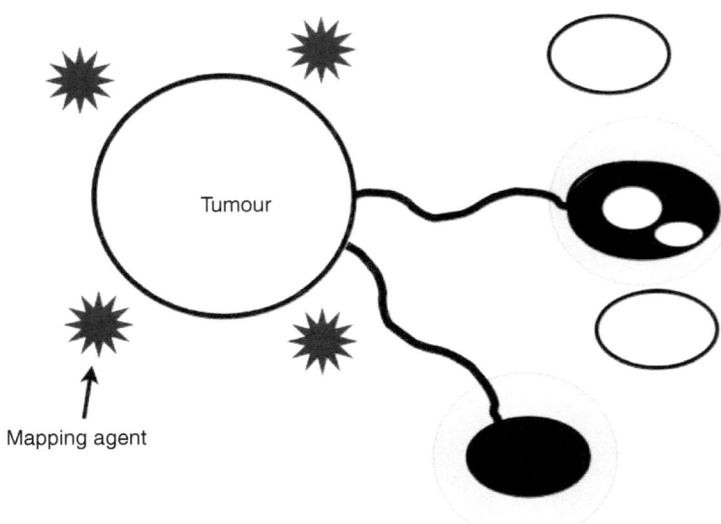

Fig. 5.2 The sentinel node concept accepts the orderly progression of metastases from the primary site to the regional draining lymph nodes. This orderly progression is defined by mapping lymphatics with dye or radioactive tracers (mapping agents) injected at the primary site. Sentinel node biopsy, in contrast to elective neck dissection, is based on the actual and not the theoretical distribution of lymphatic spread for the individual tumour. The concept recognizes diverse and variable patterns of lymphatic drainage as multiple draining lymphatic pathways in parallel arrays as opposed to 'skip metastases'

molecular studies. This is the greatest advantage of the sentinel node technique. Bivalving a lymph node, the routine practice after clearance of a neck dissection, is estimated to sample 1/1000 of the available lymph node tissue [40]. In 25 % of routine histopathologically classified N0 necks, one or more occult metastases are missed [41]. The sentinel node technique identifies patients with previously unidentified micrometastases and, therefore, improves pathological staging [42, 43].

A number of observational studies have shown that the technique is feasible in SCC of the oral cavity [44]. The validation of the sentinel concept in mucosal malignancy of the head and neck requires reliable and consistent detection of the sentinel node with the intention of identifying patients with early metastatic disease. The measurement that allows a determination of the success rate of this procedure is the false-negative rate. The false-negative rate is calculated by dividing the number of patients with a false-negative test (truly-positive) by the total number of patients with positive disease (true-positive and false-negative). Ross et al. reported the results of the first international conference on sentinel lymph node biopsy and mucosal head and neck cancer in 2002 [45]. Results from 22 centres and 360 necks were compiled. A success rate of 301/316 (95 %) was reported with a false-negative rate of 9.5 %. Stoeckli et al. reported similar findings from the second international conference [46]. The success rate was 366/379 cases from 20 centres, with a false-negative rate of 9.6 %. A prospective trial in six European centres studied sentinel lymph node biopsy in T1, T2, N0 tumours of the oral cavity and oral pharynx [47]. The patients ($n = 227$) underwent sentinel lymph node biopsy either alone or followed by elective neck dissection. Upstaging occurred in 42 (34 %) initially staged N0 by the standard histopathological technique. The false-negative rate was 7.1 %. The results of a prospective cooperative group trial of 25 institutions in North America were recently reported by Civantos and co-workers [48]. This study reported on the validation of the sentinel lymph node concept in 141 oral cancer patients staged T1, T2 and N0. The false-negative rate was 9.8 % (4/41).

The false-negative rate appears to be too high and variable to accept sentinel lymph node biopsy as a replacement for elective neck dissection at present. The following themes are common to the above series. Experience plays an important part in the success of the technique. Ross et al. Indicated that the false-negative rate was 43 % in series reporting less than 10 cases and 6.5 % in series reporting more than ten cases [45]. In most series, problems tend to occur with tumours of the floor of mouth when compared with the oral tongue [45, 48]. The head and neck represents a complex nodal basin. The techniques for sentinel lymph node biopsy were developed for less complex and more readily accessible lymph node basins in the groin and/or axilla.

The operative definition of a sentinel node is a blue (or hot) node identified within 10–15 min of injection of blue dye, and from 3 to 24 h after injection of a radiocolloid. Irrespective of this technical definition, the sentinel lymph node is the first lymph node to receive anatomical lymphatic drainage from the tumour. Blue dye is considered by many to be the gold standard for sentinel lymph node detection, as it can be identified visually in afferent lymphatics leading to the sentinel node. The problem in the head and neck is that the dye clears rapidly from the sentinel lymph node within 10–15 min. When blue dye is used alone, it is impossible to ensure that all sentinel lymph nodes have been identified. In the head and neck, it is simply not possible and/or practical because of time limitations during dissection; i.e. it takes too long to identify all possible areas of lymphatic drainage. It is not surprising that the initial experience with blue dye alone in the head and neck was not successful [49, 50]. Radionucleotide accumulates in the sentinel lymph node over a period of hours. Radionucleotide and a hand-held gamma probe facilitate sentinel lymph node biopsy by focusing the dissection with incisions placed over the 'hot spot'. Dissection can then be directed by the probe to the hot sentinel node. The radionucleotide tracer within the sentinel node can provide immediate confirmation of its identity and can be used to verify that all sentinel nodes have been removed. The technique is, however, limited by background scatter or shine-through. This results in overlapping fields of radioactivity when the sentinel lymph node is in close proximity to the primary site, such as occurs with tumours of the floor of mouth. In addition, radioactivity can pass through the sentinel node to second and third echelon nodes in a regional node basin. Therefore, not all radioactive lymph nodes are the sentinel node and the hottest node is not necessarily the sentinel lymph node. This labelling of second echelon lymph nodes is variable and dependent on numerous factors, including anatomical site, rate and volume of injection, timing of the sentinel lymph node relative to the injection, and size of particles injected [44, 51]. More sentinel lymph nodes are biopsied with radiocolloid compared with the use of dye alone. Careful evaluation during static and dynamic lymphoscintography studies done prior to the biopsy procedure has been helpful in offsetting this particular problem.

In conclusion, problems with the sentinel lymph node concept, as applied to the head and neck, are both tumour-related and technical. The tumour-related factors include the complex lymphatic anatomy and the fact that the sentinel lymph node is often close to the primary. In addition, if the sentinel lymph node is completely replaced by tumour, it will not pick up the radiocolloid. Technical factors include the time sensitivity of the blue dye and the poor spatial resolution and non-specific node labelling seen with radionucleotide. It is the authors' opinion that technical improvements will be necessary before this technique can be applied widely to the head and neck.

Summary

The incidence of occult metastases for T1 and T2 oral cancers is >20 %. Elective surgical treatment of the neck is indicated. The standard of care is a selective neck dissection tailored to the primary site, done on the basis of the predicted pattern of lymphatic drainage. Sentinel lymph node mapping targets the appropriate lymph nodes for a detailed pathological examination based on the actual pattern of lymphatic drainage. Sentinel lymph node biopsy or sentinel node-assisted elective neck dissection may provide better treatment and staging of the N0 neck than elective neck dissection alone. The fact still remains that elective neck dissection, or the use of a sentinel node-assisted elective neck dissection, will still over-treat the majority of N0 patients. Sentinel lymph node biopsy as a staging tool is minimally invasive and yields minimal morbidity. The false-negative rate is currently too high for this technique to be used for oral cancer. Technical improvements will be necessary for this technique to replace elective neck dissection.

References

1. Pitman K, Johnson J, Myers E. Effectiveness of selective neck dissection for management of the clinically negative neck. *Arch Otolaryngol Head Neck Surg* 1997;**123**:917–22.
2. Byers RM, El-Naggar AK, Lee YY, *et al.* Can we detect or predict the presence of occult nodal metastases in patients with squamous carcinoma of the oral tongue? *Head Neck* 1998;**20**:138–44.
3. Shah JP. Patterns of cervical lymph node metastasis from squamous carcinomas of the upper aerodigestive tract. *Am J Surg* 1990;**160**:405–9.
4. Yuen AP, Wei WI, Wong YM, *et al.* Elective neck dissection versus observation in the treatment of early oral tongue carcinoma. *Head Neck* 1997;**19**:583–8.
5. Vandenbrouck C, Sancho-Garnier H, Chassagne D, *et al.* Elective versus therapeutic radical neck dissection in epidermoid carcinoma of the oral cavity. Results of a randomized clinical trial. *Cancer* 1980;**46**:386–90.

6. Fakih AR, Rao RS, Borges AM, *et al.* Elective versus therapeutic neck dissection in early carcinoma of the oral tongue. *Am J Surg* 1989;**158**:309–13.
7. Gourin CG, Conger BT, Porubsky ES, *et al.* The effect of occult nodal metastases on survival and regional control in patients with head and neck squamous cell carcinoma. *The Laryngoscope* 2008;**118**:1191–4.
8. Woolgar JA, Rogers SN, Lowe D, *et al.* Cervical lymph node metastasis in oral cancer: The importance of even microscopic extracapsular spread. *Oral Oncology* 2003;**39**:130–7.
9. Andersen PE, Cambronero E, Shaha AR, *et al.* The extent of neck disease after regional failure during observation of the No neck. *Am J Surg* 1996;**172**:689–91.
10. Jess RH, Barkley HT Jr, Lindberg RD, *et al.* Cancer of the oral cavity. Is elective neck dissection beneficial? *Am J Surg* 1970;**120**:505–8.
11. Northrop M, Fletcher GH, Jesse RH, *et al.* Evolution of neck disease in patients with primary squamous cell carcinoma of the oral tongue, floor of mouth, and palatine arch, and clinically positive neck nodes neither fixed nor bilateral. *Cancer* 1972;**29**:23–30.
12. van den Brekel MW, Catelijns JA, Snow GB. Imaging of cervical lymphadenopathy. *Neuroimaging Clin N Am* 1996;**6**:417–34.
13. O'Brien CJ, Lauer CS, Fredricks S, *et al.* Tumor thickness influences prognosis of T1 and T2 oral cavity cancer—but what thickness? *Head Neck* 2003;**25**:937–45.
14. Bryne M. Is the invasive front of an oral carcinoma the most important area for prognostication? *Oral Dis* 1998;**4**:70–7.
15. Nason RW, Castillo NB, Sako K, *et al.* Cervical node metastases in early squamous cell carcinoma of the floor of the mouth: Predictive value of multiple histopathological parameters. *World J Surg* 1990;**14**:606–9.
16. Cheng A, Schmict BL. Management of the No neck in oral squamous cell carcinoma. *Oral Maxillofacial Surg Clin N Am* 2008;**20**:477–97.
17. Kligerman J, Lima RA, Soares JR, *et al.* Supraomohyoid neck dissection in the treatment of T1/T2 squamous cell carcinoma of oral cavity. *Am J Surg* 1994;**168**: 391–4.
18. Lydiatt DD, Robbins KT, Byers RM, *et al.* Treatment of stage I and II oral tongue cancer. *Head Neck* 1993;**15**:308–12.
19. Haddadin KJ, Soutar DS, Oliver RJ, *et al.* Improved survival for patients with clinically T1/T2, No tongue tumors undergoing a prophylactic neck dissection. *Head Neck* 1999;**21**: 517–25.
20. Dias FL, Kligerman J, Matos De Sa G, *et al.* Elective neck dissection versus observation in stage I squamous cell carcinomas of the tongue and floor of the mouth. *Otolaryngol Head Neck Surg* 2001;**125**:23–9.
21. Capote A, Escorial V, Munoz-Guerra MF, *et al.* Elective Neck Dissection in early-stage oral squamous cell carcinoma—does it influence recurrence and survival? *Head Neck* 2007;**29**: 3–11.
22. Huang SF, Kang CJ, Lin CY, *et al.* Neck treatment of patient with early stage oral tongue cancer. *Cancer* 2008;**112**:1066–75.
23. Nason RW, Sako K, Beecroft WA, *et al.* Surgical management of squamous cell carcinoma of the floor of the mouth. *Am J Surg* 1989;**158**:292–5.
24. Nason R, El-Sayed A, Cooke A, *et al.* Management of cervical lymph node metastases in squamous cell carcinoma of the head and neck. *Current Oncology* 1996;**3**:92–7.
25. Ferlito A, Rinaldo A, Suarez O. Often-forgotten father of functional neck dissection (in the non-Spanish-speaking literature). *Laryngoscope* 2004;**114**:1177–8.
26. Bocca E, Pignataro O, Oldini C, *et al.* Functional neck dissection: An evaluation and review of 843 cases. *Laryngoscope* 1984;**94**:942–5.
27. Medina JE, Byers RM. Supraomohyoid neck dissection: Rationale, indications, and surgical technique. *Head Neck* 1989;**11**:111–22.
28. Lindberg R. Distribution of lymph node metastases from squamous cell carcinoma of the upper respiratory and digestive tracts. *Cancer* 1972;**29**:1446–9.
29. Shah JP, Medina JE, Shaha AR, *et al.* Cervical lymph node metastasis. *Curr Probl Surg* 1993;**30**:1–335.

30. Byers RM. Modified neck dissection. A study of 957 cases from 1970 to 1980. *Am J Surg* 1985;**150**:414–21.
31. Kowalski LP, Magrin J, Waksman G, *et al.* Supraomohyoid neck dissection in the treatment of head and neck tumors. Survival results in 212 *cases. Arch Otolaryngol Head Neck Surg* 1993;**119**:958–63.
32. McGuirt WF Jr, Johnson JT, Myers EN, *et al.* Floor of mouth carcinoma. The management of the clinically negative neck. *Arch Otolaryngol Head Neck Surg* 1995;**121**:278–82.
33. Spiro RH, Morgan GJ, Strong EW, *et al.* Supraomohyoid neck dissection. *Am J Surg* 1996;**172**:650–3.
34. Fletcher GH, Jess RH Jr. Proceedings: Irradiation management of squamous cell carcinomas of the oral cavity. *Proc Natl Cancer Conf* 1972;**7**:137–42.
35. Leemans CR, Snow GB. Is selective neck dissection really as efficacious as modified radical neck dissection for elective treatment of the clinically negative neck in patients with squamous cell carcinoma of the upper respiratory and digestive tracts? *Arch Otolaryngol Head Neck Surg* 1998;**124**:1042–4.
36. Brazilian Head and Neck Cancer Study Group. Results of a prospective trial on elective modified radical classical versus supraomohyoid neck dissection in the management of oral squamous carcinoma. *Am J Surg* 1998;**176**:422–7.
37. Spiro RH, Gallo O, Shah JP. Selective jugular node dissection in patients with squamous carcinoma of the larynx or pharynx. *Am J Surg* 1993;**166**:399–402.
38. Byers RM, Weber RS, Andrews T, *et al.* Frequency and therapeutic implications of 'skip metastases' in the neck from squamous carcinoma of the oral tongue. *Head Neck* 1997;**19**:14–19.
39. Robbins KT, Shaha AR, Medina JE, *et al.,* Committee for Neck Dissection Classification, American Head and Neck Society. Consensus statement on the classification and terminology of neck dissection. *Arch Otolaryngol Head Neck Surg* 2008;**134**:536–8.
40. Krag DN. Minimal access surgery for staging regional lymph nodes: The sentinel-node concept. *Curr Probl Surg* 1998;**35**:951–1016.
41. van den Brekel MW, van der Waal I, Meijer CJ, *et al.* The incidence of micrometastases in neck dissection specimens obtained from elective neck dissections. *Laryngoscope* 1996;**106**:987–91.
42. Ross GL, Soutar DS, MacDonald DG, *et al.* Improved staging of cervical metastases in clinically node-negative patients with head and neck squamous cell carcinoma. *Ann Surg Oncol* 2004;**11**:213–18.
43. Stoeckli SJ, Alkureishi LW, Ross GL. Sentinel node biopsy for early oral and oropharyngeal squamous cell carcinoma. *Eur Arch Otorhinolaryngol* 2009;**266**:787–93. Epub 2009 Mar 21.
44. Nason RW, Torchia MG, Morales CM, *et al.* Dynamic MR lymphangiography and carbon dye for sentinel lymph node detection: A solution for sentinel lymph node biopsy in mucosal head and neck cancer. *Head Neck* 2005;**27**:333–8.
45. Ross GL, Shoaib T, Soutar DS, *et al.* The first international conference on sentinel node biopsy in mucosal head and neck cancer and adoption of a multicenter trial protocol. *Ann Surg Oncol* 2002;**9**:406–10.
46. Stoeckli SJ, Pfaltz M, Ross GL, *et al.* The second international conference on sentinel node biopsy in mucosal head and neck cancer. *Ann Surg Oncol* 2005;**12**:919–24. Epub 2005 Sep 19.
47. Ross GL, Soutar DS, Gordon MacDonald D, *et al.* Sentinel node biopsy in head and neck cancer: Preliminary results of a multicenter trial. *Ann Surg Oncol* 2004;**11**:690–6. Epub 2004 Jun 14.
48. Civantos FJ, Zitsch RP, Schuller DE, *et al.* Sentinel lymph node biopsy accurately stages the regional lymph nodes for T1–T2 oral squamous cell carcinomas: Results of a prospective multi-institutional trial. *J Clin Oncol* 2010;**28**:1395–1400. Epub 2010 Feb 8.
49. Shoaib T, Soutar DS, Prosser JE, *et al.* A suggested method for sentinel node biopsy in squamous cell carcinoma of the head and neck. *Head Neck* 1999;**21**:728–33.
50. Pitman KT, Johnson JT, Brown ML, *et al.* Sentinel lymph node biopsy in head and neck squamous cell carcinoma. *Laryngoscope* 2002;**112**:2101–13.
51. Torchia MG, Nason R, Danzinger R, *et al.* Interstitial MR lymphangiography for the detection of sentinel lymph nodes. *J Surg Oncol* 2001;**78**:151–7.

Current Options and Controversies in Reconstruction of the Oral Cavity

Ravi Sachidananda and S. Mark Taylor

Reconstruction of oral defects has always posed a challenge to the reconstructive surgeon. The ever-increasing complexity of the defects, the need for restoring form and function, and changing treatment philosophies have increased the complexity of reconstruction. Reconstructive options have evolved significantly over the past three decades. In the 1980s, pedicle flaps were the mainstay of reconstruction. However, with the introduction of free flaps, reconstructive options have increased. Technological advances and improved experience with free flaps have enhanced the success rate to 95–100 % [1, 2]. Refinements in flap insetting and advances in other related specialties have led to an overall better quality of life for the patient. This chapter summarizes the current reconstructive options and discusses the major controversies in oral reconstruction.

The goals of oral cavity reconstruction are to replace lost tissue with soft tissue, bone or both, and to optimize oral function. Oral cavity defects, for pragmatic reasons, can be classified into defects of the mucosa, mucosa and bone, bone alone and composite defects. The principles of reconstructive surgery are used to deal with these defects (Table 6.1). The surgeon should be familiar with all the available reconstructive options and utilize the best option taking into consideration the defect size, patient co-morbidity and the impact of reconstruction on the overall long-term quality of life of the patient.

R. Sachidananda
Head & Neck Surgery and Microvascular Reconstruction,
QE2 HSC, VG Site, 3044 Dickson Building, 5820 University Avenue,
Halifax, NS B3H 1 V7, Canada
e-mail: entravi@yahoo.com

S.M. Taylor (✉)
Otolaryngology, Head & Neck Surgery, Facial Plastic and Reconstructive surgery,
QE2 HSC, VG Site, 3044 Dickson Building, 5820 University Avenue,
Halifax, NS B3H 1 V7, Canada
e-mail: smtaylorwashu@yahoo.com

© The Author(s) 2012
K.A. Pathak, R.W. Nason (eds.), *Controversies in Oral Cancer*,
Head and Neck Cancer Clinics, DOI 10.1007/978-81-322-2574-4_6

Table 6.1 Reconstructive ladder

Options in head and neck reconstruction
Healing by secondary intention
Primary closure
Skin grafting
Local flaps
Pedicle flaps
Free tissue transfer
Obturators

Reconstructive Options for Covering Mucosal Defects

Primary Closure/Healing by Secondary Intention

Small defects of the oral cavity can be closed by primary closure. This is a good option for small defects of the oral tongue, buccal mucosa and the floor of the mouth. With respect to tongue defects, a resection involving ≤30 % of the tongue can be closed primarily without significantly affecting speech or swallow [3]. Hsiao et al. have recommended tongue reconstruction when the resection involves >50 % of the tongue [4, 5]. With increased defect size, patients were often unable to lift the tongue tip and had poor tongue-to-palate contact, resulting in premature spilling of the bolus into the pharynx. They also noted large amounts of stasis in the floor of the mouth and prolongation of oral transit time.

Healing by secondary intention is an option often considered for early cancers of the tongue, floor of the mouth, buccal mucosa and hard palate after transoral laser surgery. Although it is good for dynamic areas, such as the palate, it may cause tethering in more dynamic areas, such as the tongue. The senior author (SMT) has considerable experience with transoral laser microsurgery and prefers healing by secondary intention for T1 lesions of the tongue and floor of the mouth in situations in which opposing healing surfaces between the tongue and floor of the mouth are absent, which will lead to secondary scarring and tethering of the tongue.

Skin Grafting

Skin grafting can be used for a variety of defects involving the oral cavity. The graft can be obtained from the groin or axilla with minimal donor site morbidity. The graft needs to be sutured to the defect with a bolster dressing to give a watertight closure. Bolsters often necessitate a tracheostomy to protect the airway. The results of skin grafting have been excellent, with Schramm and Myers reporting 97 % complete healing rates [6]. Recently, Girod et al. reported better results with the use of acellular dermis grafting [7]. This graft reconstruction gives a more natural-appearing mucosal surface, and comparable, if not superior, functional status. The main disadvantages of skin grafting are scar contracture and the lack of bulk.

Locoregional Flaps

Local flaps have been used for reconstruction of limited intraoral defects. The limited arc of rotation and donor site morbidity are the main constraints. Three flaps described below need special mention.

Nasolabial Flaps

Nasolabial flaps are cutaneous flaps based on the facial artery and are generally used for small to intermediate defects of the oral cavity. They can be used either as a superiorly based flap or as an inferiorly based flap. The superiorly based flap is utilized mainly for closing small maxillary and buccal mucosal defects, whereas the inferiorly based flap is used to close floor of the mouth defects [8, 9]. These flaps have generally provided good functional results [10]. A modification of this flap as a myocutaneous flap has been described [11]. Although survival of the flap is good, significant upper lip weakness usually remains, causing cosmetic deformity. The main drawback of this flap is the need for a second surgery to divide the flap and transfer hair-bearing skin, especially in males.

Infrahyoid Myocutaneous Flap

This flap was originally described by Wang and Shen in 1980 [12]. More recently, it has been gaining popularity in selected patients who are not ideal candidates for free-flap reconstruction. The flap is based on the superior thyroid artery and is used mainly in moderate-sized defects of the oral cavity (floor of the mouth, retromolar trigone and buccal mucosa). In the original technique, the complication rate was high (47 %), and was thought to be related to poor venous drainage [13]. A recent modification, as described by Dolivet, has increased the success rate of the flap to ~100 % [14, 15]. The main contraindications for the flap are previous neck dissection, history of thyroid surgery and the presence of N3 nodal disease.

Pectoralis Major Myocutaneous Flap

Pectoralis major myocutaneous flap (PMMF) is the 'workhorse pedicle flap' for intraoral reconstruction. This flap is reliable, versatile and close to the head and neck region. Generally, the donor site can be closed primarily with little donor site morbidity. The flap is based on the pectoral branch of the thoracoacromial artery. Although free tissue transfer remains the gold standard for reconstruction of oral cavity defects, recent studies have shown changing trends in the indications for PMMF in oral reconstruction (Table 6.2) [16, 17]. The main shortcomings are the limited arch of rotation and the tendency for partial necrosis (4–29 %) of the skin paddle resulting in high complication rates (36–63 %) [18–21]. In addition, tethering of the tongue may occur due to the bulky nature of the flap and a tendency to sag downwards, often limiting its use in the reconstruction of glossectomy defects. At our centre, we have preferred to use the myofascial pectoralis major flap in an attempt to reduce flap bulk and to eliminate the possibility of skin flap-related complications [16].

Table 6.2 Current indications for reconstruction with pectoralis major myocutaneous flap in oral cavity defects

Indications
Co-morbidity
Vessel-depleted neck
Salvage flap
Recurrent disease
Covering exposed palate
Composite and complex defects
Paucity of resources

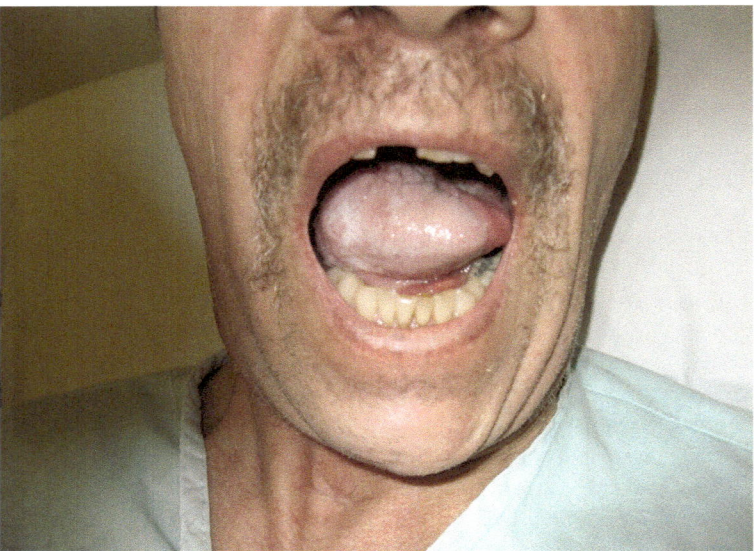

Fig. 6.1 Hemiglossectomy defect resurfaced with radial forearm flap

Free Flaps

Radial Forearm Flap (Fig. 6.1)

The radial forearm free flap remains the workhorse of intraoral reconstruction because of its pliability, thinness and ease of harvest. The flap is based on the radial artery and the two venae comitantes that accompany it. It can also be based on the superficial system incorporating either the cephalic vein or the basilic vein.

This flap offers unparalleled versatility in oral reconstruction. It can be harvested to a considerable size to include the whole arm, and a segment of bone can be harvested (radius) if an osseous component is needed. A bi-lobed design can be used to reconstruct the floor of the mouth and tongue to prevent tethering [22]. The flap can be de-epithelialized and folded or harvested with additional subcutaneous fat to add bulk [23]. It can also be used for resurfacing full-thickness defects involving skin, muscle and mucosa. The flap can be asensate if the medial or lateral antebrachial nerve is used for sensory innervation [24].

The main drawback of this flap is donor site-related problems, such as poor healing of the skin graft, cosmesis and, rarely, functional deficits. Transfer of hair-bearing skin to the oral cavity may also pose a problem. However, if the patient receives radiotherapy, hair follicles are often destroyed by treatment.

Anterolateral Flap

Although the radial forearm flap remains the gold standard for soft-tissue reconstruction of the oral cavity, it has limitations when a large skin paddle is needed for reconstruction. It often leaves behind unsightly scars leading to poor cosmetic outcome. This has led to the popularization of the anterolateral thigh flap, which has replaced the radial forearm flap in some centres as the first choice in oral reconstruction [25].

The anterolateral thigh flap was described originally as a septocutaneous flap by Song et al. in 1984 [26]. It is now popular as a musculocutaneous perforator artery flap based on the descending branch of the lateral circumflex artery and its two venae comitantes. Its use in head and neck reconstruction was popularized largely by Wei et al. and the reported success rate has been between 95 and 97 % [25–27]. The main advantage is its adaptability in covering almost any soft tissue defect in the oral cavity. The flap can be thinned to resurface hemiglossectomy defects, or it can be used as a myocutaneous flap with the vastus lateralis whenever additional bulk is required (total glossectomy). Further, it can be used as a folded flap to resurface through-and-through defects of the oral cavity. The flap can also be used as a split double paddle based on two perforators (chimaeric flap) for resurfacing more complex defects. This versatility of both design and composition in addressing almost any defect makes the anterolateral thigh flap popular for intraoral reconstruction [28, 29].

Donor site morbidity is low given that the donor site can be closed primarily. Also, careful dissection and preservation of the nerve to the vastus lateralis decreases quadriceps weakness. Recently, it has been demonstrated that even in instances in which the vastus has been harvested, donor site morbidity is very low [27]. The only limitation is the thickness of subcutaneous fat in the Caucasian population, which may preclude its use where thin pliable flaps are needed. A site-specific anatomical approach to oral cavity reconstruction is given in Table 6.3.

Table 6.3 Preferred reconstructive options based on site-specific anatomical defects

Defect site	Main option	Alternatives
Hemiglossectomy	RFF	ALT
Total glossectomy	ALT	Modified RFF Rectus/latissimus PMMF
Floor of mouth	Radial forearm	Nasolabial IMF
Buccal mucosa	Radial forearm	Nasolabial Temporoparietal
Mandible	Free fibular	Iliac crest Scapular system
Maxilla	Free fibular	Scapular system

ALT anterolateral thigh flap, *IMF* infrahyoid myocutaneous flap, *PMMF* pectoralis major myocutaneous flap, *RFF* radial forearm flap

Reconstruction of Bony Defects

Segmental defects of the mandible often create considerable cosmetic and functional deficits of the oral cavity. Historically, reconstruction of the mandible has been attempted with many techniques, such as free bone grafts, metallic and alloplastic materials, or with a combination of a metallic reconstruction plate with vascularized muscle. None of these methods have stood the test of time, mainly because of complications and the inability to withstand radiation. Mandibular reconstruction has been revolutionized by the introduction of a free fibular flap (Figs. 6.2 and 6.3). This flap, based on the peroneal artery and the two venae comitantes, provides excellent bone stock and length to make it the first choice for bony reconstruction of mandibular and maxillary defects. The success rate has been shown to be between 92 and 100 % [2, 30, 31]. The length and the predictable blood supply enables multiple osteotomies for recreating complex areas of the mandible (arch/condyle) or maxilla (palate). The main disadvantage is the unreliability and non-pliable nature of the skin paddle, and the inability to use the flap in patients with significant peripheral vascular disease.

Scapular flaps are a group of versatile flaps often used in the head and neck region for reconstruction of both maxillary and mandibular defects [32]. These flaps are based on the circumflex scapular vessels, with the option of extending to the subscapular vessels if additional pedicle length is needed. It is possible to elevate a uni- or bipaddled flap with bone when the need arises to reconstruct complex 3-dimensional defects of the maxilla or mandible. Its main shortfalls are the inability to use the two-team approach and thin bone stock, precluding the use of osseo-integrated implants. Presently, its use is limited to patients who need complex

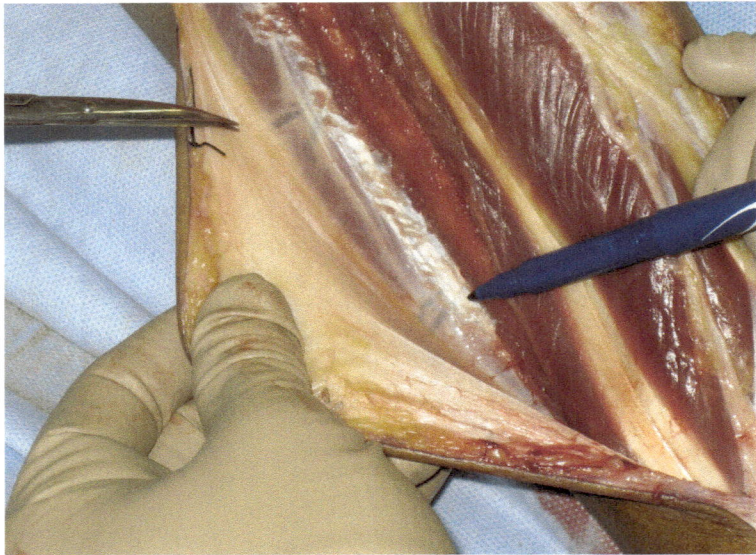

Fig. 6.2 Free fibular flap with skin perforators

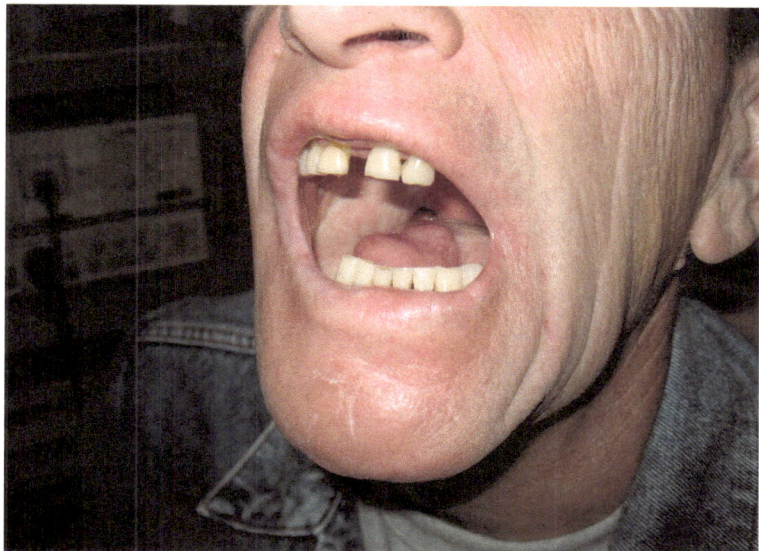

Fig. 6.3 Free fibular osseocutaneous flap for lateral mandibular defect

reconstruction of the oral cavity, facial skeleton and overlying facial skin or for those who are known to have peripheral vascular disease.

The iliac crest free flap is a composite flap based on the deep circumflex iliac artery and the two venae comitantes [32]. This flap can be used in situations in which both bone and bulk are needed for reconstruction. A good stock of cancellous bone and the natural curvature of the bone resembling the mandible make it a good choice for reconstruction of the arch of the mandible and for osseo-integrated implants. The main limitations are the short pedicle, significant donor site morbidity (pain, hernia, meralgia paraesthetica) and the thickness of the skin paddle, which often limits its use in the reconstruction of composite defects.

Controversies in Oral Reconstruction

The availability of an array of reconstructive options and the ever-increasing refine-ments in surgery have stimulated debate over the choice of techniques, their impact on functional outcomes and overall cost implications. We perceive the following as the main areas of debate in oral reconstruction:

- The role of sensate flaps in improving function
- The functional superiority of free flap reconstruction compared with a palatal obturator in closing palatomaxillary defects
- The choice of flap (free versus locoregional)
- Utility of a plate flap option in lateral mandibular reconstruction.

Does Sensate Flap Reconstruction Improve Oral Cavity Functional Outcomes?

The ability to sense food is a prerequisite for chewing, swallowing, and preventing drooling and pooling of saliva. This aspect of functional restoration was first attempted by David et al. when they used the innervated deltopectoral flap for oral reconstruction [33]. Since then, several attempts have been made to restore normal function by utilizing sensate flaps. For example, Santamaria et al. reported that the sensory recovery of the innervated radial forearm flap in tongue reconstruction provided sensory abilities to near normal levels [34]. Kurialose et al. reported that sensate radial forearm flaps had sensation superior to that of the donor site skin and approached that of the normal functioning tongue [24]. A detailed study by Boyd et al. compared the functional outcome of patients who underwent reconstruction with a sensate radial forearm flap with non-sensate flaps [35]. All the patients who underwent the procedure were subjected to detailed sensory testing to evaluate touch, two-point discrimination, pressure and temperature. The results were compared with non-innervated radial forearm flaps and PMMFs. The authors concluded that innervated flaps were superior to non-innervated flaps in all the modalities of sensation tested, almost approaching that of the normal tongue. They also found that patients who had innervated flaps had a greater degree of perception of food in the mouth compared to that of controls.

Kimata et al. extended this concept to other flaps (sensate anterolateral flaps and sensate rectus abdominal flaps) [36]. Their study confirmed the findings of improved sensation in innervated flaps compared with the non-innervated flap cohort. Further, they found that sensory recovery is often influenced by the type of anastomosis (sensory nerve to sensory nerve). For example, the antebranchial cutaneous nerve to lingual nerve or inferior alveolar nerve provided better results compared with sensory to motor nerve anastomosis.

Re-innervation of the sensate flap occurs in the following two patterns: (i) Through peripheral ingrowth from the surrounding nerves, and (ii) through the surgically created neural pathway. In non-innervated flaps, sensory recovery occurs solely through peripheral ingrowth, rendering almost one-third of the patients completely anaesthetized over the flap region [37]. This is additionally influenced by other factors that may impair the ingrowth of nerve fibres (e.g. radiation and composite flap harvest). Although these studies have demonstrated that sensory recovery occurs faster in innervated flaps, evidence is still scarce to show clearly that benefits gained by sensate flaps actually translate into superior functional results. Two recent papers have attempted to evaluate the influence of sensate flaps on speech intelligibility, mastication and swallowing [38, 39]. Loewen et al. compared sensate radial forearm free flaps in tongue reconstruction with healthy controls and found that speech intelligibility and mastication may still be impaired despite the use of a sensate flap [38]. Biglioli et al. compared the results of a 'sensate' radial forearm flap with a 'non-sensate' flap and found better speech intelligibility with sensate flaps and no significant benefit in swallowing [39].

To summarize, evidence shows that innervated flaps hasten sensory recovery. However, what is still not known is the extent of benefit of a sensate flap on functional domains, such as mastication, speech and swallow in oral reconstruction.

Reconstruction of Hard Palate Defects: Reconstruct or Obturate?

Resecting an oral cancer of the palate results in connection of the oral and nasal cavities. This defect affects speech, swallow, dentition and cosmesis. Traditionally, restorations of such defects were accomplished by palatal prosthesis. Although this was ideal for small defects, it failed in large defects because of hyper-nasality and reflux of fluid contents into the nasal cavity [40]. Also, long-term prosthetic care is needed, as poor care often results in malodour and crusting. Furthermore, reliance on the prosthesis for simple tasks, such as speech and swallowing, requires a degree of manual dexterity for everyday use. This has led to the evaluation of other forms of rehabilitation, including free flaps and osseointegrated implants.

Palato-maxillary defects have been standardized by using several classifications. These classifications take into account the various components of the mid face (horizontal and vertical bony components, soft tissue, and the extent of orbital and zygomatic resection). Okay et al. have proposed a defect-oriented classification for functional reconstruction of the palato-maxillary defect [41]. This describes an array of techniques incorporating both surgical and prosthetic rehabilitation.

On the basis of the Okay system of classification, most defects that are class 1A, 1B and some class 2 defects can be rehabilitated successfully with an obturator (Table 6.4). The prosthesis is generally stable and well tolerated [41]. With increasing defect size, there is loss of dentition and supporting bony arch, leading to instability of the prosthesis. These require free vascularized bone grafts for support and further prosthodontic rehabilitation.

Rogers et al. compared the health-related quality of life between an obturator and free flap in maxillary reconstruction [42]. The study reported that both modalities of treatment gave similar quality-of-life benefits. When oral symptoms were evaluated specifically, patients with an obturator were self-conscious and less satisfied with upper dentures. They also reported problems with the obturator in terms of leakage of food into the nasal cavity and soreness in the mouth. An example of a free fasciocutaneous forearm flap for a class 1 maxillary defect is seen in Fig. 6.4.

The main drawback of the study was that the group of patients treated with obturators had a smaller resection of the palato-maxillary region. Genden et al. compared the functional and quality-of-life outcomes in patients who had class 2 defects [43]. These patients were either rehabilitated with an obturator or a vascularized bone-containing free flap. They found that patients who underwent free-tissue transfer with vascularized bone had better functional outcomes with respect to speech and mastication, and an overall better quality of life without significant donor site morbidity. Other important factors that determine the failure rate of the obturation

Table 6.4 Okay classification for reconstruction of palato-maxillary defects [41]

Defect type	Extent of defect	Reconstruction
Class 1A	Defect involving hard palate but not tooth-bearing alveolus	Obturator Local flaps Fasciocutaneous free flap
Class 1 B	Defect involving pre-maxilla or any portion of maxillary alveolus and dentition posterior to canines	Obturator Fasciocutaneous flap
Class 2	Defects involving any portion of hard palate and tooth-bearing maxillary alveolus and only one canine. Anterior margin within pre-maxilla. Includes transverse palatectomy defects of <50 % of hard palate	Obturator Osseocutaneous free flap
Class 3	Defects involving any portion of hard palate and tooth-bearing alveolus, including both canines. Includes total and transverse palatectomy defects of >50 % of hard palate	Osseocutaneous free flap

Class 1a   Class 1b   Class 1b

Class 2   Class 2

Class 3   Class 3   Class 3

include the degree of resection of the palate (>25 % of palate), previous radiotherapy and inclusion of the soft palate in the resection [44, 45].

In summary, patients with small palatal defects can be rehabilitated with obturators, whereas larger defects require free flaps to close the communication between

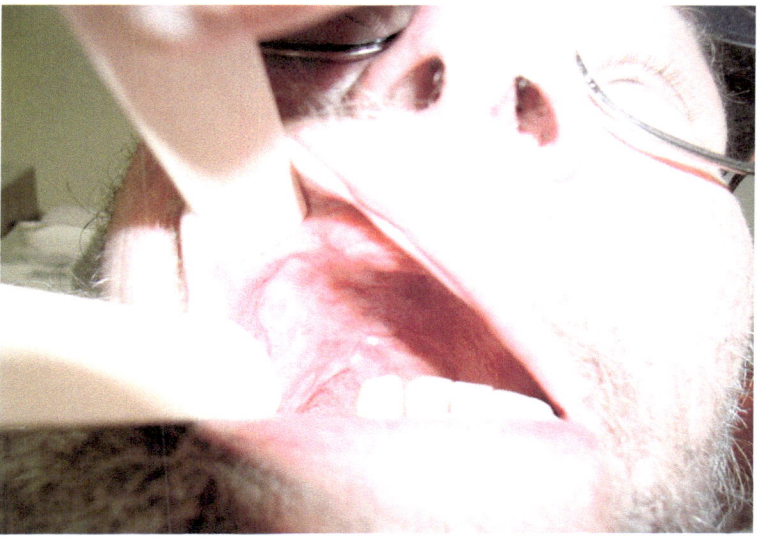

Fig. 6.4 Class 1 defect reconstructed with radial forearm flap

the oral and nasal cavities. As a general principle, our group prefers free osteocutaneous flaps, specifically the free fibular flap, in patients in whom the resection involves half or more of the hard palate or in resections that involve both canines. The decision should be taken in the context of the patient's personal choice, the state of oral dentition and the general physical status of the patient.

Pedicled Flap Versus Free Flaps in Soft Tissue Defects of the Oral Cavity

With advances in microvascular reconstruction, the success rate of free tissue transfer has risen to ~95 % and has mostly replaced pedicled flaps as the first choice for intra-oral reconstruction. This excessive reliance on free flaps in oral reconstruction has been questioned. Using a free flap increases operative time, manpower, resources and the cost of surgery with no clear evidence of functional benefit over a pedicled flap.

Although locoregional flaps (tongue flaps, nasolabial flaps, PMMF) have tissue characteristics similar to the tongue/oral mucosa, they are often limited by factors such as donor site morbidity, poor vascularity (radiotherapy), limited arc of rotation, tethering and distortion of the oral cavity. One of the commonly used regional flaps in oral reconstruction is the PMMF. Although the risk of total flap necrosis in PMMF is low (2–3 %), the reported overall complication rate of PMMF is high [18, 19, 46]. This is related mainly to partial necrosis of the skin paddle leading to wound breakdown and fistula formation. The poor vascularity can be explained by the nature of the relationship between the skin paddle and the vascular pedicle (perpendicular in oral reconstruction). Further, plication of the flap and cramping of the bulky paddle in patients with an intact mandibular arch leads to compromised vascularity at the periphery of the skin paddle and high complication rates [47].

One of the common sites for oral reconstruction is resurfacing of glossectomy defects. This is resurfaced most commonly with a free radial forearm flap. The thin and pliable nature of the tissue makes it an ideal tissue match. Further, the option of sensory reinnervation with the lateral antebrachial cutaneous nerve enables the design of sensate flaps to hasten sensory recovery. When a larger bulk is needed, as in total glossectomy defects, other options, such as the anterolateral thigh flap or a rectus abdominis/latissumus flap can be used.

Presently, the success rate of free flap reconstruction is ~95 %; with increasing experience and good monitoring a success rate of almost 100 % can be reached. With most flaps having a long pedicle and a diameter of at least 2 mm, the chance of vascular complications has decreased significantly. This makes free flaps the first choice of reconstruction in oral cancer.

The overall cost is an important factor in microvascular reconstruction, with some authors questioning the choice of free flap as a cost-effective procedure [48, 49]. Earlier studies have reported a longer operative time, longer stay in the ICU, and the significantly high cost of free flap reconstruction. These studies have focused primarily on costs incurred during hospitalization for surgery. Two case–control studies have evaluated the cumulative cost incurred over a length of time (1–2 years) and found no significant overall cost benefit in using a pedicled flap over a free flap [50, 51].

Although many studies have compared the cost-effectiveness of pedicled flaps over free flaps, literature evaluating the functional superiority of a free flap compared with a pedicled flap is scarce. Su et al. compared the functional outcomes of the radial forearm flap with that of the PMMF in reconstruction of the oral tongue [52]. They found that patients who underwent reconstruction with a radial forearm flap had a higher speech intelligibility rating than those with pedicled flap reconstruction in cases of both hemiglossectomy and total glossectomy. Swallowing outcomes were similar in both groups. Other studies have used G tube dependence as an indirect measure of functional outcomes and found higher G tube dependence in patients who underwent a PMMF flap compared with a free flap [53].

Free flaps have now replaced pedicled flaps as the choice for oral reconstruction in moderate to large defects of the oral cavity. With increasing experience and good monitoring techniques, the success rate of free flaps is consistently >95 %. Presently, pedicled flaps are more or less limited to small defects of the oral cavity or to patients with significant co-morbidity or for reconstructive salvage.

Reconstruction of the Mandible: Is There a Role for a Plate Flap Option?

Vascularized bone containing free flaps is the gold standard for mandibular reconstruction. In reconstruction of large composite defects of the mandible, it is recognized that the soft tissue component may have limitations in resurfacing complex

Table 6.5 Outcomes of study with plate flap option in mandibular defects

Author	Year	No of patients	Complications (%)	Follow up (months)	Conclusion
Irish et al. [54]	1995	51	24	48	Complications higher if >3 mandibular regions resected
Blackwell et al. [55]	1996	15	40	7–15	Abandon
Arden et al. [56]	1999	31	45	37	Avoid if resection >5 cm
Blackwell and Lacombe [57]	1999	27	7	19	Need long-term follow up
Shpitzer et al. [58]	2000	57	19	12	Acceptable in selected patients
Wei et al. [59]	2002	80	69	22	Not a good option
Head et al. [60]	2003	210	8	26	Reasonable alternative
Poli et al. [61]	2003	25	33	60	Acceptable in selected patients
Okura et al. [62]	2005	100	38	60	Avoid in irradiated patients
Chepeha et al. [63]	2008	40	10	60	Acceptable in selected patients
Coletti et al. [64]	2009	110	36	14	Abandon

3-dimensional defects. To overcome this, several authors have either used more than one flap for reconstruction or a bridging plate with a free flap. Patients with large composite defects often have advanced stage disease with significant co-morbidity, limiting the use of more than one flap. A bridging plate and flap may be used for reconstruction of such defects.

A review of the literature has highlighted considerable controversy in the utility of plates in lateral mandibular reconstruction (lateral to the mandibular canine tooth), with some authors completely abandoning the procedure and some using it selectively (Table 6.5). This is due mainly to the significant hardware-related complications, such as fracture of the plate, loosening of screws and exposure of the plate. Further, secondary salvage procedures are necessary, either to remove the hardware or to reconstruct with bone or soft tissue flaps should complications arise [59].

Blackwell et al. reported their initial experience with 15 patients who underwent primary reconstruction of lateral mandibular defects using soft-tissue free flaps combined with a first-generation THORP plate [55]. Their initial experience showed a 33 % complication rate associated with the plates, which occurred within 15 months. The same group later reported excellent results using the second-generation reconstruction plate [57, 60]. This study compared the efficacy of the plate flap option with free vascularized bone grafts in a large series of patients. Of the 210 patients undergoing reconstruction for lateral mandibular defects, 151 patients underwent vascularized bone grafts and 59 patients had a combination of soft tissue flap and a bridging plate. They reported success rates of 94 % within the bone graft group and 92 % within the plate flap group (success defined as restoration of mandibular continuity). Most of the flap-related complications in the bone graft group occurred early, whereas the plate flap group showed late complications (extrusions and plate fractures). They attributed their success to superior hardware stability offered by the second-generation THORP plates and to limiting the use of plates to short segmental lateral defects.

The second-generation THORP plate (locking plate) generally has reduced hardware-related complications. The AO reconstruction plates (bridging plates) are non-locking. When non-locking screws are tightened, pressure is translated through the plate to the underlying bone, leading to bone resorption beneath the plate, causing the plate to loosen. The second-generation THORP plates are superior as they offer stability, which is independent of contact between the plate under-surface and the bone. Further, they have a lower profile and threaded screw heads that screw into the plate to lock it; the plate–screw complex acts as a single functional unit, minimizing pressure transmission to the bone [64].

In addition to plate geometry, many tissue factors influence plate failure. These include altered masticatory vectors after bone loss, decreased vascularity at the alloplastic interface and loss of tissue volume, which increases dead space [56]. Tissue contracture and fibrosis over the plate often result in plate exposure. This problem has been overcome by Chepeha et al. by using the so-called 'compartment approach' in reconstruction of lateral mandibular defects, whereby these surgeons essentially 'over reconstruct' the volume of lost tissue with revascularized soft tissue over a plate, thus preventing contraction of the skin over the plate [63]. Whereas this approach leads to a reduction of plate exposure rate from 38 to 8 %, the technique does not reduce the plate fracture rates.

Thirty-one patients with oral cancer were reviewed retrospectively by Arden et al. [56] These patients were treated with composite resection and reconstruction with bridging plates. All patients were irradiated; an overall complication rate of 45 % was reported. The complication rate was 81 % for defects >5 cm and 7 % for defects <5 cm. A similar study by Irish et al. on 51 patients who underwent mandibular reconstruction with the THORP plate followed over a 4-year period reported a 24 % complication rate [54]. The incidence of complications was higher for patients who had >3 mandibular regions resected. Long-term studies by Okura et al. in a large series of patients reported a 62 % overall success rate after 5 years [62]. They also found that anterolateral defects and preoperative radiotherapy adversely affected plate success [62].

Reconstruction of lateral mandibular defects with a bridging plate and a soft tissue free flap is a reasonable option in selected patients who require a large volume of pliable soft tissue reconstruction with short segmental bony defects. This should be considered in the context of anticipated plate-related morbidity over the years.

Conclusion
Reconstruction of the oral cavity is deceptively complex. In spite of a wide variety of available options, it is often impossible to replicate the complex functioning of the oral cavity. The ultimate goal of reconstruction is to maximize functional potential by utilizing the best currently available options for reconstruction. It is possible that in the years to come, advances in stem cell research, allotransplantation and osteosynthesis may play a larger role in restoring both form and function.

References

1. Suh JD, Sercarz JA, Abemayor E, *et al*. Analysis of outcome and complications in 400 cases of microvascular head and neck reconstruction. *Arch Otolaryngol Head Neck Surg* 2004;**130**:962–6.
2. Cordeiro PG, Disa JJ, Hidalgo DA, *et al*. Reconstruction of the mandible with osseous free flaps: A 10-year experience with 150 consecutive patients. *Plast Reconstr Surg* 1999;**104**:1314–20.
3. McConnel FM, Pauloski BR, Logemann JA, *et al*. Functional results of primary closure vs flaps in oropharyngeal reconstruction: A prospective study of speech and swallowing. *Arch Otolaryngol Head Neck Surg* 1998;**124**:625–30.
4. Hsiao HT, Leu YS, Chang SH, *et al*. Swallowing function in patients who underwent hemi-glossectomy: Comparison of primary closure and free radial forearm flap reconstruction with videofluoroscopy. *Ann Plast Surg* 2003;**50**:450–5.
5. Hsiao HT, Leu YS, Lin CC. Primary closure versus radial forearm flap reconstruction after hemiglossectomy: Functional assessment of swallowing and speech. *Ann Plast Surg* 2002;**49**:612–16.
6. Schramm VL Jr, Myers EN. Skin grafts in oral cavity reconstruction. *Arch Otolaryngol* 1980;**106**:528–32.
7. Girod DA, Sykes K, Jorgensen J, *et al*. Acellular dermis compared to skin grafts in oral cavity reconstruction. *Laryngoscope* 2009;**119**:2141–9.
8. Lazaridis N, Tilaveridis I, Karakasis D. Superiorly or inferiorly based 'islanded' nasolabial flap for buccal mucosa defects reconstruction. *J Oral Maxillofac Surg* 2008;**66**:7–15.
9. al Khabori MJ, Natarajan B, Thomas M, *et al*. Naso-labial flap in the reconstruction of floor of the mouth defects. *J Laryngol Otol* 1993;**107**:320–3.
10. Hofstra EI, Hofer SO, Nauta JM, *et al*. Oral functional outcome after intraoral reconstruction with nasolabial flaps. *Br J Plast Surg* 2004;**57**:150–5.
11. Burkey BB, Coleman JR Jr. Current concepts in oromandibular reconstruction. *Otolaryngol Clin North Am* 1997;**30**:607–30.
12. Wang HS, Shen JW, Ma DB, *et al*. The infrahyoid myocutaneous flap for reconstruction after resection of head and neck cancer. *Cancer* 1986;**57**:663–8.
13. Magrin J, Kowalski LP, Santo GE, *et al*. Infrahyoid myocutaneous flap in head and neck reconstruction. *Head Neck* 1993;**15**:522–5.
14. Dolivet G, Gangloff P, Sarini J, *et al*. Modification of the infra hyoid musculo-cutaneous flap. *Eur J Surg Oncol* 2005;**31**:294–8.
15. Ricard AS, Laurentjoye M, Faucher A, *et al*. 276 cases of horizontal infrahyoid myocutaneous flap. *Rev Stomatol Chir Maxillofac* 2009;**110**:135–7. Epub 2009 Apr 28. French.
16. Ethier JL, Trites J, Taylor SM. Pectoralis major myofascial flap in head and neck reconstruction: Indications and outcomes. *J Otolaryngol Head Neck Surg* 2009;**38**:632–41.
17. Liu HL, Chan JY, Wei WI. The changing role of pectoralis major flap in head and neck reconstruction. *Eur Arch Otorhinolaryngol* 2010. Epub ahead of print.
18. Mehta S, Sarkar S, Kavarana N, *et al*. Complications of the pectoralis major myocutaneous flap in the oral cavity: A prospective evaluation of 220 cases. *Plast Reconstr Surg* 1996;**98**:31–7.
19. Shah JP, Haribhakti V, Loree TR, *et al*. Complications of the pectoralis major myocutaneous flap in head and neck reconstruction. *Am J Surg* 1990;**160**:352–5.
20. Liu R, Gullane P, Brown D, *et al*. Pectoralis major myocutaneous pedicled flap in head and neck reconstruction: Retrospective review of indications and results in 244 consecutive cases at the Toronto General Hospital. *J Otolaryngol* 2001;**30**:34–40.
21. Kasler M, Banhidy FG, Trizna Z. Experience with the modified pectoralis major myocutaneous flap. *Arch Otolaryngol Head Neck Surg* 1992;**118**:931–2.
22. Uwiera T, Seikaly H, Rieger J, *et al*. Functional outcomes after hemiglossectomy and recon-struction with a bilobed radial forearm free flap. *J Otolaryngol* 2004;**33**:356–9.
23. Haughey BH, Taylor SM, Fuller D. Fasciocutaneous flap reconstruction of the tongue and floor of mouth: Outcomes and techniques. *Arch Otolaryngol Head Neck Surg* 2002;**128**:1388–95.

24. Kuriakose MA, Loree TR, Spies A, *et al*. Sensate radial forearm free flaps in tongue reconstruction. *Arch Otolaryngol Head Neck Surg* 2001;**127**:1463–6.
25. Wei FC, Jain V, Celik N, *et al*. Have we found an ideal soft-tissue flap? An experience with 672 anterolateral thigh flaps. *Plast Reconstr Surg* 2002;**109**:2219–26.
26. Song YG, Chen GZ, Song YL. The free thigh flap: A new free flap concept based on the septocutaneous artery. *Br J Plast Surg* 1984;**37**:149–59.
27. Mäkitie AA, Beasley NJ, Neligan PC, *et al*. Head and neck reconstruction with anterolateral thigh flap. *Otolaryngol Head Neck Surg* 2003;**129**:547–55.
28. Chana JS, Wei FC. A review of the advantages of the anterolateral thigh flap in head and neck reconstruction. *Br J Plast Surg* 2004;**57**:603–9.
29. Ali RS, Bluebond-Langner R, Rodriguez ED, *et al*. The versatility of the anterolateral thigh flap. *Plast Reconstr Surg* 2009;124 (6 Suppl):e395–407.
30. Shpitzer T, Neligan PC, Gullane PJ, *et al*. Oromandibular reconstruction with the fibular free flap. Analysis of 50 consecutive flaps. *Arch Otolaryngol Head Neck Surg* 1997;**123**:939–44.
31. Hidalgo DA, Pusic AL. Free-flap mandibular reconstruction: A 10-year follow-up study. *Plast Reconstr Surg* 2002;**110**:438–49; discussion 450–1.
32. Takushima A, Harii K, Asato H, *et al*. Choice of osseous and osteocutaneous flaps for mandibular reconstruction. *Int J Clin Oncol* 2005;**10**:234–42.
33. David DJ. Use of an innervated deltopectoral flap for intraoral reconstruction. *Plast Reconstr Surg* 1977;**60**:377–80.
34. Santamaria E, Wei FC, Chen IH, *et al*. Sensation recovery on innervated radial forearm flap for hemiglossectomy reconstruction by using different recipient nerves. *Plast Reconstr Surg* 1999;**103**:450–7.
35. Boyd B, Mulholland S, Gullane P, *et al*. Reinnervated lateral antebrachial cutaneous neurosome flaps in oral reconstruction: Are we making sense? *Plast Reconstr Surg* 1994;**93**:1350–9; discussion 1360–2.
36. Kimata Y, Uchiyama K, Ebihara S, *et al*. Comparison of innervated and non-innervated free flaps in oral reconstruction. *Plast Reconstr Surg* 1999;**104**:1307–13.
37. Kerawala CJ, Newlands C, Martin I. Spontaneous sensory recovery in non-innervated radial forearm flaps used for head and neck reconstruction. *Int J Oral Maxillofac Surg* 2006;**35**:714–17. Epub 2006 May 11.
38. Loewen IJ, Boliek CA, Harris J, *et al*. Oral sensation and function: A comparison of patients with innervated radial forearm free flap reconstruction to healthy matched controls. *Head Neck* 2010;**32**:85–95.
39. Biglioli F, Liviero F, Frigerio A, *et al*. Function of the sensate free forearm flap after partial glossectomy. *J Craniomaxillofac Surg* 2006;**34**:332–9. Epub 2006 Jul 21.
40. Gillespie CA, Kenan PD, Ferguson BJ. Hard palate reconstruction in maxillectomy. *Laryngoscope* 1986;**96**:443–4.
41. Okay DJ, Genden E, Buchbinder D, *et al*. Prosthodontic guidelines for surgical reconstruction of the maxilla: A classification system of defects. *J Prosthet Dent* 2001;**86**:352–63.
42. Rogers SN, Lowe D, McNally D, *et al*. Health-related quality of life after maxillectomy: A comparison between prosthetic obturation and free flap. *J Oral Maxillofac Surg* 2003;**61**:174–81.
43. Genden EM, Okay D, Stepp MT, *et al*. Comparison of functional and quality-of-life outcomes in patients with and without palatomaxillary reconstruction: A preliminary report. *Arch Otolaryngol Head Neck Surg* 2003;**129**:775–80.
44. Irish J, Sandhu N, Simpson C, *et al*. Quality of life in patients with maxillectomy prostheses. *Head Neck* 2009;**31**:813–21.
45. Rieger JM, Wolfaardt JF, Jha N, *et al*. Maxillary obturators: The relationship between patient satisfaction and speech outcome. *Head Neck* 2003;**25**:895–903.
46. Milenovic A, Virag M, Uglesic V, *et al*. The pectoralis major flap in head and neck reconstruction: First 500 patients. *J Craniomaxillofac Surg* 2006;**34**:340–3. Epub 2006 Jul 24.

47. Mallet Y, El Bedoui S, Penel N, *et al.* The free vascularized flap and the pectoralis major pedicled flap options: Comparative results of reconstruction of the tongue. *Oral Oncol* 2009;**45**:1028–31. Epub 2009 Sep 30.
48. Tsue TT, Desyatnikova SS, Deleyiannis FW, *et al.* Comparison of cost and function in reconstruction of the posterior oral cavity and oropharynx. Free vs pedicled soft tissue transfer. *Arch Otolaryngol Head Neck Surg* 1997;**123**:731–7.
49. McCrory AL, Magnuson JS. Free tissue transfer versus pedicled flap in head and neck reconstruction. *Laryngoscope* 2002;**112**:2161–5.
50. de Bree R, Reith R, Quak JJ, *et al.* Free radial forearm flap versus pectoralis major myocutaneous flap reconstruction of oral and oropharyngeal defects: A cost analysis. *Clin Otolaryngol* 2007;**32**:275–82.
51. Funk GF, Karnell LH, Whitehead S, *et al.* Free tissue transfer versus pedicled flap cost in head and neck cancer. *Otolaryngol Head Neck Surg* 2002;**127**:205–12.
52. Su WF, Hsia YJ, Chang YC, *et al.* Functional comparison after reconstruction with a radial forearm free flap or a pectoralis major flap for cancer of the tongue. *Otolaryngol Head Neck Surg* 2003;**128**:412–18.
53. Chepeha DB, Annich G, Pynnonen MA, *et al.* Pectoralis major myocutaneous flap vs revascularized free tissue transfer: Complications, gastrostomy tube dependence, and hospitalization. *Arch Otolaryngol Head Neck Surg* 2004;**130**:181–6.
54. Irish JC, Gullane PJ, Gilbert RW, *et al.* Primary mandibular reconstruction with the titanium hollow screw reconstruction plate: Evaluation of 51 cases. *Plast Reconstr Surg* 1995;**96**:93–9.
55. Blackwell KE, Buchbinder D, Urken ML. Lateral mandibular reconstruction using soft-tissue free flaps and plates. *Arch Otolaryngol Head Neck Surg* 1996;**122**:672–8.
56. Arden RL, Rachel JD, Marks SC, *et al.* Volume-length impact of lateral jaw resections on complication rates. Arch *Otolaryngol Head Neck Surg* 1999;**125**:68–72. PubMed
57. Blackwell KE, Lacombe V. The bridging lateral mandibular reconstruction plate revisited. *Arch Otolaryngol Head Neck Surg* 1999;**125**:988–93.
58. Shpitzer T, Gullane PJ, Neligan PC, *et al.* The free vascularized flap and the flap plate options: Comparative results of reconstruction of lateral mandibular defects. *Laryngoscope* 2000;**110**:2056–60.
59. Wei FC, Celik N, Yang WG, *et al.* Complications after reconstruction by plate and soft-tissue free flap in composite mandibular defects and secondary salvage reconstruction with osteocutaneous flap. *Plast Reconstr Surg* 2003;**112**:37–42.
60. Head C, Alam D, Sercarz JA, *et al.* Microvascular flap reconstruction of the mandible: A comparison of bone grafts and bridging plates for restoration of mandibular continuity. *Otolaryngol Head Neck Surg* 2003;**129**:48–54.
61. Poli T, Ferrari S, Bianchi B, *et al.* Primary oromandibular reconstruction using free flaps and thorp plates in cancer patients: A 5-year experience. *Head Neck* 2003;**25**:15–23.
62. Okura M, Isomura ET, Iida S, *et al.* Long-term outcome and factors influencing bridging plates for mandibular reconstruction. *Oral Oncol* 2005;**41**:791–8.
63. Chepeha DB, Teknos TN, Fung K, *et al.* Lateral oromandibular defect: When is it appropriate to use a bridging reconstruction plate combined with a soft tissue revascularized flap? *Head Neck* 2008;i**30**:709–17.
64. Coletti DP, Ord R, Liu X. Mandibular reconstruction and second generation locking reconstruction plates: Outcome of 110 patients. *Int J Oral Maxillofac Surg* 2009;**38**:960–3. Epub 2009 May 6.

Challenges in Preserving Salivary Gland Functions

7

Rashmi Koul and Arbind Dubey

Introduction

Challenges in the field of oncology include not only improving success rates of current cancer therapies, but also reducing the morbidity associated with successful treatment modalities. For instance, preserving the function of the salivary glands in patients undergoing radiation for head and neck cancer (HNC) is challenging, but the question is how to achieve this. This chapter explores techniques for preserving salivary gland function in patients undergoing radiation for oral cancers.

Radiation, used either as a primary or secondary therapeutic modality, often results in significant morbidity in HNC, which adversely affects a patient's quality of life [1]. Radiation invariably results in salivary gland dysfunction. This is one of the most common and agonizing side-effects and remains with the patient throughout his or her life [2].

Saliva is a frothy, watery substance produced in and secreted by the salivary glands. Human saliva is composed of 98 % water, the other 2 % consisting of other compounds, such as electrolytes, antibacterial material, mucus and some enzymes. The salivary enzymes break down some of the starch and fat in food, as well as the food lodged in the teeth, thus protecting them from bacterial tooth decay. Saliva also lubricates and protects the oral cavity. Whereas the amount of saliva produced in a healthy person per day is debatable, estimates range from 0.75 to 1.5 L per day; it is generally accepted that during sleep saliva production drops to almost zero. In humans, the submandibular gland contributes 70–75 % of the secretion, and the parotid gland secretes 20–25 %; small amounts are secreted from the other salivary glands. Any condition that affects salivary production results in xerostomia [3].

R. Koul (✉) • A. Dubey
Department of Radiation Oncology, University of Saskatchewan,
Staff Radiation Oncologist, Allan Blair Cancer Centre, 4101 Dewdney Ave,
Regina, SK S4T7T1, Canada
e-mail: rkoul@cancercare.mb.ca

© The Author(s) 2012
K.A. Pathak, R.W. Nason (eds.), *Controversies in Oral Cancer*,
Head and Neck Cancer Clinics, DOI 10.1007/978-81-322-2574-4_7

Xerostomia

Xerostomia can cause difficulty in speech, mastication, swallowing and deglutition. The patient loses protective remineralization of enamel, which predisposes to cavities, caries and other oral infections. The oral mucosa becomes dry, cracked and painful. Patients have low tolerance for dental prostheses because of tissue friability and lack of lubrication. Swallowing patterns may also be abnormal, in that movement of a bolus from the mouth to the pharynx is slowed [4].

Radiation-induced xerostomia arises secondary to acute degeneration and necrosis of serous cells within 24 h of radiation to both the parotid and submandibular glands. The histopatholoigical changes occur within 10–12 weeks after completing radiation therapy. Loss of serous acini, distortion of ducts and aggregation of plasma cells and lymphocytes are predominant. Mucous cells are less affected. Glands become fibrotic and get filled with dense collagen 6 months later. Precisely how this inflammation eventually causes damage to the parenchymal cells is uncertain. The salivary function continues to decline throughout a typical course of treatment and may become barely measurable at the end of 7 weeks' treatment. The decreased flow is accompanied by increased salivary viscosity, decreased pH, increased concentration of sodium, chloride, calcium and magnesium, and decreased amounts of bicarbonates and immunoglobulin A (IgA). Xerostomia usually persists for several years; patients may or may not recover from it, depending on the volume of gland radiated, total dose and patient variation [5]. So, the most effective way of preserving salivary function is primary prevention.

Treatment Considerations

Literature from the West is replete with strategies for preserving salivary gland function in patients undergoing radiation for oral cancers. Unfortunately, there is no consensus on the choice of method, its cost-effectiveness, and comparisons to evaluate outcome. Popular strategies include the use of amifostine, intensity-modulated radiation therapy (IMRT) to spare the parotid glands and surgery for sparing the salivary glands. These modalities have met with varying degrees of success. Currently, the most effective methods in use are meticulous radiation treatment planning to spare >50 % of the salivary glands and surgical sparing of the salivary glands [6]. However, in the absence of phase III randomized and prospective data, the superiority of one technique over the other cannot be proved. Physicians treating this site have to understand the caveats of each modality before deciding which one will provide optimal benefit to the patient.

Conformal Radiation Techniques

Radiation techniques have changed and improved considerably over the past decade or so. In the early 1990s, with the introduction and popularization of 3-dimensional (3-D) conformal radiation, each patient received customized treatment fields according to their anatomy. However, this technique was not perfect as clinicians were unable to effectively carve out normal organs (such as the salivary glands) from high-radiation dose areas. Treatment planning systems have evolved and treatment delivery systems have caught up with modern technology. These enhancements in radiation oncology have emerged as powerful tools to deliver tumoricidal doses to cancerous tissues while simultaneously protecting normal tissues, especially salivary function. The therapeutic ratio has improved significantly. This planning and radiation delivery capability has been achieved by IMRT. IMRT is an advanced mode of high-precision radiotherapy (RT) that utilizes computer-controlled linear accelerators to deliver precise radiation doses to a malignant tumour or specific areas within the tumour.

IMRT allows for the radiation dose to conform more precisely to the 3-D shape of the tumour by modulating or controlling the intensity of the radiation beam in multiple small volumes. IMRT also allows higher radiation doses to be focused on regions within the tumour while minimizing the dose to the surrounding normal critical structures. Treatment is carefully planned by using 3-D computed tomography (CT) scan images of the patient in conjunction with the computerized dose. The ability to fuse images, such as with positron emission tomography (PET) and MRI, helps to delineate the tumour on the basis of anatomy and metabolic activity, and has led to better precision. IMRT offers an excellent tool that optimizes the therapeutic ratio by maximizing tumour dose and minimizing radiation to normal tissue by applying complex computer algorithms. This technique is particularly popular because of its precise delivery system and hence it has become the standard of practice in most cancer institutions.

Sufficient recent data are now available to highlight the fact that parotid gland sparing by IMRT in HNC patients improves xerostomia-related quality of life compared with conventional radiation, both at rest and during meals. However, inconsistencies are evident in terms of the strength of the correlation between patient-reported xerostomia and the measured salivary output. This correlation has not been consistently reported in studies [7]. Looking at the correlation coefficients in these studies, salivary flow rates alone could not be responsible for the variability in scores [8]. Kam et al. reported a similar pattern with salivary flow rates significantly better after IMRT compared with 2-dimensional RT. This did not correlate with patient-reported xerostomia scores [9]. This could be due to failure of adequate data collection in terms of patient-reported symptoms or because sparing of the parotid glands alone was not sufficient. Similar results were reported in another study randomizing patients with early-stage nasopharyngeal cancer to IMRT or to 3-D RT. The parotid saliva is devoid of mucins and is responsible for failure of the preserved parotid saliva to impact greatly on patient-reported xerostomia [10].

Mucin is a mucosal lubricant and helps maintain a hydrated state due to its ability to bind water and as a result give a sense of hydration. It also acts as a selective permeability barrier. Mucin-secreting glands, such as the minor salivary glands, produce <10 % of the total volume of saliva but contribute the majority of the total mucins [11]. Submandibular glands are also a source of mucins. The importance of the mucin-producing glands in determining the severity of xerostomia was demonstrated in various studies. There was a correlation with RT doses to these glands, their salivary output, and patient-reported xerostomia. Also, studies that used surgical transfer of a submandibular gland to the non-irradiated submental space, resulted in a significant patient-reported benefit [12–14].

With the IMRT technique for bilateral neck radiation, dose reduction to the contralateral submandibular gland is difficult, owing to its close proximity to the jugulodigastric nodes, which are the first-echelon nodes in most HNCs and require high doses of radiation. Partial sparing of the parotid glands using IMRT results in preservation of the parotid salivary flow rates, but only modest improvement in patient-reported xerostomia [15]. The issue of sparing of the mucin-producing salivary glands has not yet been resolved. Munter and colleagues reported on a series of 18 patients who received IMRT and required bilateral neck irradiation. Their goals were to spare the parotid glands without any increase in local failure rates, and to analyse functional changes in the salivary glands as a function of radiation dose using quantitative scintigraphy. The target mean dose for the parotid glands was 26 Gy, which was achieved in one gland in 11 of 18 patients and in both glands in 5 patients. The team made no attempt to spare the submandibular glands; they used scintigraphy to measure salivary gland function. With maximal uptake as the primary measurement parameter, a dose threshold of 30 Gy was observed for induction of xerostomia [16]. However, this did not correlate with the Radiation Therapy Oncology Group (RTOG) score, which measures subjective clinical symptoms. In patients receiving IMRT, the incidence of late RTOG grade 2 xerostomia was 17 % [16]. In a series of 23 patients, Parliament et al. used a stricter criterion of goal mean dose to one parotid of <20 Gy [7]. The actual combined mean dose to both parotids was 30 Gy. Oral health and quality of life was measured using the University of Washington instrument [18]. Interestingly, patients with better preserved, unstimulated salivary flow rates tended to report lower xerostomia scores [17].

In contrast to the many publications on treating adult patients with IMRT, data on the use of IMRT in the paediatric population is limited. Bhatnagar et al. have reported a favourable outcome with IMRT used to treat 22 children [18]. They described substantial sparing of surrounding critical structures in cranial, abdominopelvic or spinal lesions, which altogether constitute very difficult oncological situations. Conventional treatment technologies would have resulted in a markedly higher dose to the organs at risk or would have required a compromise of the possible target dose. Penagaricano et al. summarized their experience of five children treated with IMRT with a high degree of conformality [19]. The dose distribution could be adapted to arc-shaped volumes in contrast to conventional therapy in which treated volumes are usually box-shaped and encompass big areas of treated normal tissue. Similar conclusions have been drawn by Paulino et al. in their synopsis of this method for children [20]. They conclude that IMRT is a valuable alternative to conventional treatment techniques for paediatric cancer patients. The improved dose distribution coupled with the ease of delivery of the IMRT fields make this technique very attractive, especially in view of the potential to increase local control and possibly improve survival. A third survey of a heterogeneous group of children treated with IMRT has been described by Teh et al. within a general article about decreased treatment-related morbidity with IMRT [21]. Experiences with 185 patients treated with IMRT, including 40 children suffering from different tumours, have been presented. In keeping with the conclusions drawn by various authors using IMRT in the studies described above, Teh et al. also concluded that IMRT offers new options in escalating the dose and achieving better local control while simultaneously reducing toxicity. Apart from compilations of composed cohorts, a larger number of articles provide data on special indications and more predefined collectives. They deal especially with intracranial or head and neck tumours, because the sensitive structures such as eyes, brainstem, parotid glands and inner ears represent an extraordinary challenge for radiotherapeutic management [22, 23]. Penagaricano et al. showed that even if the entire craniospinal axis is irradiated, as required in medulloblastoma or germinoma, this can be done with improved conformity and sparing of sensitive structures [24]. In a retrospective planning evaluation, they illustrate the possibilities of helical tomotherapy (as one solution of IMRT) to cover a target volume of this size, while simultaneously avoiding the problems of field junctions and the resulting dangers of under- or over-dosage inherent in conventional techniques. After treating the whole craniospinal axis, the primary tumour region is supposed to be irradiated with an extra boost to the posterior fossa. Huang et al. describe reduced ototoxicity when sparing the inner ear by IMRT compared with conventional RT, in which the cochlear region receives the full therapeutic dose [23]. Thirteen percent of the IMRT group had grade 3 or 4 hearing loss, compared with 64 % of the conventional RT group. The sparing of the hearing apparatus is of special importance, as several modern, combined chemotherapy regimens contain ototoxic agents, such as cisplatinum. Jain et al. showed that this improvement in ototoxicity was not achieved at the cost of increased neuropsychological changes [25].

Another challenging situation is that IMRT might substantially improve the treatment of retinoblastoma. Krasin et al. presented a planning study comparing different conventional photon, electron and IMRT techniques in the treatment of intraocular retinoblastoma [26]. The best sparing of the bony orbit was achieved with IMRT, yielding a promising potential of avoiding asymmetrical bone growth after successful RT. The mean volume of bony orbit treated with IMRT >20 Gy (as a threshold of bone growth disturbance) was 60 % in contrast to 90 % by conventional techniques. Schroeder et al. reported on 22 children with localized intracranial ependymomas treated with IMRT [27]. They were able to achieve a 3-year local control of 68 % while enabling minimal rates of toxicity (no visual or hearing impairment, no necrosis and no myelitis). In summary, available data suggest that using IMRT to keep the mean dose of the parotid glands to ≤26 Gy decreases the risk of long-term xerostomia. Furthermore, data suggest that sparing the submandibular and, perhaps, minor salivary glands can decrease this risk further. Therefore, in patients receiving IMRT, the parotid, submandibular and submental glands should be contoured and preserved as much as possible.

Surgery: Salivary Gland Transfer

Another means of preserving salivary gland function is the surgical manipulation of the salivary glands before embarking on radiation. Jha et al. successfully demonstrated prevention of xerostomia by surgical transfer of the submandibular salivary gland to the submental space before starting radiation therapy. In this study, surgery was the prime modality of management, followed by adjuvant postoperative radiation treatment. The most recent update of this study had 84 patients, 76 of whom were evaluable. The median follow up was 14 months. Of the 60 patients with salivary gland transfers, 43 patients had surgery for the primary and postoperative radiation treatment with protection of the transferred salivary gland. For these 43 patients, results of prevention of xerostomia at various intervals after radiation treatment were recorded. At the end of radiation treatment, 81 % of the patients had none or minimal xerostomia and 19 % developed moderate to severe xerostomia. Surgical transfer was relatively simple and added 45 min to the surgical procedure. No complications were attributed to the submandibular gland transfer but patients' appraisal and satisfaction with current function were not evaluated [28].

Recently, immense emphasis has been place on quality-of-life measurement in clinical trials. Being subjective, parameters of quality of life are best measured from the patient's perspective. Recent advances in cancer treatments for locally controlling cancers of the head and neck have prompted clinicians to turn their attention to supporting and preserving their patients' quality of life. The promising results of surgical sparing of the salivary glands prompted the RTOG to introduce the 0244 phase II study to further investigate the role of submandibular gland transfer in a multi-institutional setting; the trial is currently open and is enrolling patients with biopsy-confirmed squamous cell carcinoma of the oropharynx, hypopharynx or larynx, or those having an unknown primary tumour with unilateral metastases to the neck nodes and at least 80 % of the parotids receiving $\geq$50 Gy. The choice of side for submandibular salivary gland transfer depends on the side of both the uninvolved neck and the primary tumour. The transferred salivary gland is identified with the help of CT scans taken in the treatment position. The shielding is then drawn to cover >70 % of the transferred submandibular salivary gland and the major part of the sublingual salivary glands [29]. The preliminary study results of submandibular gland transfer look promising. This surgical procedure may improve the quality of life and health of many HNC patients after radiation therapy [30]. Clinical trials to determine the advantages of the procedure and its effect on other health outcomes, particularly long-term survival, are ongoing.

Pharmacological Considerations

Whereas concomitant delivery of chemotherapy and RT appear to have a synergistic effect on tumour control, this strategy also has potential disadvantages. As treatment regimens become more aggressive, the risk of normal tissue injury also increases, potentially resulting in treatment breaks or dose reductions that may limit the success of therapy. Thus, if the toxicity can be reduced, not only the median survival time, but also the Q-time (quality-adjusted survival time) can be improved. This analysis underlies the rationale for employing the radio protector amifostine to attempt to reduce the high rate of salivary gland suppression encountered in the promising, yet toxic, concurrent chemo-radiation regimens [31]. Amifostine

(Ethyol) is a thiophosphate prodrug that is dephosphorylated in normal tissues to its active metabolite, WR-1065. Once inside the cell, this reduced drug scavenges radiation-induced reactive oxygen species. Fortunately, amifostine levels are high in the salivary glands, and this provides a potential benefit in preventing xerostomia [32]. This effect was first reported in patients who were treated with radiation for HNC in 1990. Since then, an enormous amount of data has emerged. Data presented at the 40th American Society of Clinical Oncology meeting from a phase III randomized, clinical trial involving 303 HNC patients showed that amifostine reduced the incidence of moderate-to-severe dry mouth (xerostomia) in patients receiving radiation therapy for their disease [32]. Two years after treatment, patients treated with amifostine retained the ability to produce saliva. Further, the data showed no evidence of tumour protection for the 24-month period of the study. Tumour control, progression-free survival and overall survival at each follow-up visit were not significantly different between treatment groups [32]. Before amifostine can be applied widely in combined modality regimens, it is important to establish that no adverse interactions exist between it and cytotoxic agents. Theoretically, drug interactions between amifostine and chemotherapeutic agents are not likely to occur, as amifostine is cleared rapidly from the plasma (90 % of the drug is cleared within 6 min) [33]. The effect of amifostine on the pharmacokinetics of cisplatinum has been shown not to decrease cisplatin's pharmacokinetic parameters [34]. Koukourakis et al. reported the results of a randomized trial comparing subcutaneous amifostine with placebo in a group of 140 patients, 40 of whom had an HNC [35]. Patients were treated with RT as definitive treatment or after incomplete resection, but no specific dose–volume requirements to the salivary glands were specified. Amifostine was administered daily at a dose of 500 mg diluted in 2.5 ml of normal saline 20 min before RT. Grade 3 of 4 oral mucosal toxicities were reduced significantly with the addition of amifostine (30 % in the radiation-only arm versus 0 % in the amifostine arm; p=0.02). A non-significant reduction in the number of days during which radiation was interrupted was also seen. Treatment breaks were given to patients who demonstrated grade 3 mucositis, and treatment was interrupted until mucositis returned to grade 1. Radiation-induced xerostomia, defined here as severe mouth dryness and persistent use of water as a substitute for saliva, was noted in 75 % of patients in the RT-only arm versus 58 % of patients in the amifostine arm (p=0.32) [36].

Pilocarpine has also been tried widely by physicians in the past decade. Pilocarpine hydrochloride is a direct-acting cholinergic parasympathomimetic agent. It acts through direct stimulation of the muscarinic receptors and can have broad, widely distributed effects on smooth muscle and exocrine tissues. Pilocarpine produces increased smooth muscle tone of the gastrointestinal and genitourinary systems, eye and respiratory tract. Exocrine glands of the lacrimal, gastric, intestinal, respiratory tract and salivary systems are also affected [37]. The benefits of pilocarpine may arise from the hyper-stimulation of small residual volumes of unirradiated parotid gland. The usefulness of pilocarpine when the entirety of both parotids have been irradiated to high doses is unclear [38]. Results with pilocarpine have been inconsistent, but several investigations have demonstrated its effectiveness in reducing the rate of xerostomia when used after RT [39]. These placebo-controlled, randomized trials found that ~50 % of patients given 5–10 mg tid noted an improvement in the sensation of oral dryness. Warde and colleagues examined the use of pilocarpine during and after RT for HNC in 130 patients in a phase III placebo-controlled trial [40]. These patients began taking pilocarpine on the first day of RT and continued intake until 1 month after RT was completed. Their study found no beneficial effect of pilocarpine on xerostomia when examining a patient-completed linear analogue scale measuring the acute toxicity of RT, or a patient questionnaire measuring quality of life at 1, 3 and 6 months after completion of RT. These findings are at variance with non-randomized data from studies by Zimmerman and associates, in which patients also began pilocarpine on the first day of RT and continued its use until 3 months post-RT [41]. This study found that the use of pilocarpine was associated with significantly less subjective xerostomia than that reported by a similar cohort of patients who had not received pilocarpine (p<0.01). Unpleasant cholinergic side-effects occur in approximately half of the patients using this drug. Adverse reactions can include the following: (1) Gastrointestinal effects such as nausea, vomiting, epigastric distress, abdominal cramping and diarrhoea; (2) genitourinary effects, such as bladder tightness and urinary frequency; (3) central nervous system effects such as headache, syncope and tremors; and (4) cardiovascular effects, such as flushing, diaphoresis, hypotension, hypertension and arrhythmias. Pilocarpine therapy must be used judiciously if cardiac failure, bronchial asthma, urinary tract obstruction, peptic ulcer, gastrointestinal spasm, hyperthyroidism, or Parkinson disease are present [37]. Despite these severe side-effects and mixed results, pilocarpine continues to be administered to patients today. In many instances, patients require lifelong treatment with this drug. Therefore, these patients may experience a lifetime of extremely bothersome and possibly hazardous consequences in an attempt to relieve their xerostomia.

Cevimeline (Evoxac) is another muscarinic agonist often used for the treatment of radiation-induced xerostomia. Several studies have reported on this drug's effect on xerostomia attributable to Sjögren syndrome (SS) [42, 43]. However, trials of the drug for radiation-induced xerostomia have not been published. Fife and colleagues conducted a 6-week, randomized, double-blind, placebo-controlled study in 75 patients with SS [44]. Seventy-six percent of the patients in the 30 mg tid group reported a global improvement in their dry mouth symptoms, compared with 35 % in the placebo group. This difference was statistically significant at p=0.0043. There was no evidence that patients in the 60 mg tid group had better global evaluation scores than those in the 30 mg tid group. Although both dosages of cevimeline provided symptomatic improvement, 60 mg tid was associated with an increase in the occurrence of adverse events, particularly gastrointestinal tract disorders. A 12-week, randomized, double-blind, placebo-controlled study was conducted in 197 patients with SS by Petrone and associates [42]. Statistically significant global improvement in the symptoms of dry mouth (p=0.0004) was seen for the 30 mg tid group compared with placebo, but not for the 15 mg group, compared with placebo. Like pilocarpine, cevimeline has numerous side-effects because of its parasympathomimetic properties. These may include headache, visual disturbance, lacrimation, sweating, respiratory distress, gastrointestinal spasm, nausea, vomiting, diarrhoea, atrioventricular block, tachycardia, bradycardia, hypotension, hypertension, shock, mental confusion, cardiac arrhythmia and tremors [45]. Again, for patients to gain any relief from their xerostomia, many have to endure numerous and, at times, debilitating consequences.

Symptomatic Approaches

When pharmaceutical agents have proven to be ineffective or the side-effects become too bothersome, patients often resort to symptomatic measures to treat their xerostomia. They may choose treatment with household products, such as tap water, saline or bicarbonate solutions. These measures are simply methods for continual moistening of the oral tissues. In addition, sugarless lozenges and gums are often used and have been found to provide significant relief in some patients [46]. A study by Markovic and colleagues found that the use of a sorbitol-sweetened gum was associated with statistically significant stimulated whole-mouth and parotid salivary flow rate increases when compared with unstimulated whole-mouth and parotid salivary flow rates [47]. Commercially available mouthwashes may provide some relief by acting as moistening agents for the oral tissues. In addition, several mouthwashes have been further developed to provide antimicrobial proteins that reduce the incidence of caries in these at-risk patients. An increasingly popular option is the use of saliva substitutes, which have been developed to provide a more lasting sensation of oral wetness than the above-mentioned therapies. The substitutes usually contain a polymer based on carboxymethylcellulose, which is used as a thickening agent to provide lubrication to the oral tissues [48]. Other commercially available saliva substitutes that better simulate human saliva contain natural mucins, primarily porcine gastric mucin or bovine submandibular mucin.

Future Considerations

Research is currently being directed at developing artificial saliva that not only provides lubrication and oral moistness but, like natural human salivation, also protects against microorganisms. Development of saliva substitutes based on novel thickening agents in the hope of providing longer retention on the mucosal surface is another area of current research. Substitutes based on linseed polysaccharide (Salinum®, Miwana AB, Gallivare, Sweden) or xanthan gum polysaccharide (Xialine®, Lommerse Pharma BV, Oss, The Netherlands) have been shown to be effective in patients with SS [49]. In another study, the clinical effectiveness of the BioXtra dry-mouth care system was evaluated [50]. BioXtra has an extract of colostrum, which is the key enzyme in this innovation. BioXtra's unique formulation mimics not only the essential salivary peroxidase system, but also introduces other naturally occurring salivary components to help supplement the mouth's natural antibacterial, non-immune and immune mechanisms. The BioXtra products, based on a tried and tested patented formulation, combine salivary protective systems with colostrum extract [51]. Moreover, immunoglobulins present in the colostrum extract also bind to the isolated bacteria inhibiting re-adhesion to the epithelial cells, thereby helping to regenerate and repair damaged mucosa. The active ingredients in BioXtra, derived from milk and milk by-products, have been carefully selected to create a formula that works optimally to provide regular supplementation of essential oral components. Any ingredients known to lessen the effectiveness of the formulation have been excluded. These include, among others, sodium lauryl sulphate, sodium fluoride, alcohol and menthol [52]. In the mouth, concentrations of salivary antimicrobials can vary according to factors such as diet, stress, vitamin deficiency, ageing, medications, systemic diseases and medical treatments. In these patients, a xerostomia questionnaire consisting of three parts (xerostomia symptom score, quality-of-life survey and visual analogue scale [VAS]) was completed by 34 patients suffering from radiation-induced xerostomia before and after 4 weeks of treatment with the BioXtra moisturizing gel, toothpaste and mouthwash [53]. The BioXtra products significantly diminished the most common symptoms of xerostomia. Mean VAS score at the start of treatment was 59.8; after treatment this decreased to 36.4 (p < 0.001). Twenty-six patients (77 %) responded to treatment, 11 of whom (32 %) reported a major improvement. Quality of life significantly improved under treatment; mean QoL (quality of life) score at the start was 59.4; this increased to 70.5 (p < 0.001). None of the 34 patients reported any adverse effects and all but 1 patient found the BioXtra dry mouth-care system easy to use. The results of this study suggest that the BioXtra dry mouth-care system is effective in reducing the symptoms of radiation-induced xerostomia and improving the quality of life of xerostomia patients, even if a proportion of the benefit is due to a placebo effect [54]. Nevertheless, further research is necessary to evaluate the efficacy of BioXtra on oral health.

Anethole trithione is a bile secretion-stimulating drug, commonly known as a cholagogue. It stimulates the parasympathetic nervous system and increases the secretion of acetylcholine, resulting in the stimulation of salivation from serous acinic cells [55]. Anethole trithione has been used for many years in the treatment of chronic xerostomia, but reports differ on its efficacy. Whereas some studies report improvements in salivary flow rates in drug-induced xerostomia, trials in patients with SS show conflicting results [56]. Side-effects reported include abdominal discomfort and flatulence. Dosages of 75 mg tid may be effective in treating patients with mild-to-moderate symptoms of xerostomia, but further research is needed to establish its safety and efficacy in this setting [57].

Yohimbine is an alpha-2 adrenergic antagonist that indirectly results in an increase of cholinergic activity peripherally [58]. In one small, randomized, double-blind, crossover study, the effect of yohimbine was compared to that of anethole trithione in ten patients treated with psychotropic medications. Patients given yohimbine 6 mg tid for 5 days showed significantly increased saliva flow (p < 0.01) when compared with anethole trithione 25 mg tid [59].

Human interferon alpha (IFN-α) is currently undergoing clinical trials to determine the safety and efficacy of low-dose lozenges in the treatment of salivary gland dysfunction and xerostomia in patients with SS [60]. In one study, the therapeutic effect of IFN-α on the xerostomia of SS was determined by injecting 1×10^6 units of IFN-α intramuscularly once weekly. Saliva production was quantitated by the Saxon test. Variation in saliva production measured at monthly intervals during the 3-month period prior to administration of IFN-α was within ±0.30 g/2 min. After administration of IFN-α, saliva production increased to >0.30 g/2 min in six patients; the increase was statistically significant by the paired t-test (p = 0.002). The result suggested a beneficial effect of this agent in increasing saliva production in these patients [61].

Another area of research includes the production of antimicrobial peptides originally derived by histatins—antifungal proteins occurring naturally in the serous salivary glands. Prednisolone irrigation of the parotid glands is being investigated as a potential treatment for xerostomia in patients with SS [62].

Acupuncture may be an option for patients with xerostomia secondary to radiation therapy for head and neck malignancy. The mechanism by which acupuncture or electrical stimulation relieves xerostomia is elusive [63]. Consideration of the Eastern philosophy from which acupuncture emerges supports the representation that xerostomia is due to a blockage of qi (pronounced 'chee'). Acupuncture removes that block and restores the host to 'balance' or homoeostasis. This clearly is difficult to translate to a Western construct. Western practitioners believe parasympathetic mediation to be partly responsible, although the plethora of points and stimulation techniques make that claim tenuous and difficult to prove. Nevertheless, an emerging body of information supports acupuncture in the symptomatic relief of xerostomia secondary to head and neck irradiation. Although the most reliable acupuncture technique is currently under investigation, the studies discussed below have all shown promise. Among the more recent studies, Blom and colleagues were the first to describe the effect of acupuncture on xerostomia in patients from a large Swedish trial [64]. These authors initially conducted a trial in 38 patients. Acupuncture was delivered to 5–8 of 28 points. When analysed over the entire acupuncture population, all patients had increased flow rates at the 6-month follow-up evaluation compared with baseline. Patients continuing with acupuncture regimens subsequently had higher stimulated and unstimulated flow rates at 3 years compared with patients who had discontinued acupuncture [65].

A study published by San Diego investigators uses a much simpler auricular-based xerostomia protocol. [66] This technique involves needling three points in the bilateral ears and a single point in the distal radial aspect of the index finger. Median palliation using a subjective questionnaire (Xerostomia Inventory [XI]) was 9 points (range: 0–25 points); 35 patients (70 %) noted an improvement of ≥10 % over baseline XI values [67]. Using a cut-off of ≥10 points on the XI, 24 patients (48 %) received benefit. Duration of effect for 13 patients (26 %) exceeded 3 months [68]. An unpublished practice analysis recently evaluated the addition of the acupuncture point CV-24 (Chengjiang, unpublished data), a point located at the centre of the mentolabial groove directly below the lip. Patients treated with the previously reported acupuncture regimen with the addition of an acupuncture needle at CV-24 experienced enhanced salivation in many cases [69]. In 2003, a group from

McMaster University, Canada published the results of a phase I/II study with transcutaneous electrical nerve stimulation using a proprietary device called a codetron [70]. In this study, 37 patients who completed therapy showed statistically increased salivation using a visual analogue scale at both 3 and 6 months of follow up ($p < 0.001$ and $p < 0.0001$). Furthermore, statistically increased basal and stimulated salivation was noted at both follow-up visits [71]. Prospective, randomized trials of acupuncture for xerostomia after head and neck RT are ongoing in France and in a collaborative programme between Emory University and Memorial Sloan-Kettering Cancer Center, USA. With the results of these and other ongoing studies, the technique and understanding of the use of acupuncture for xerostomia are expected to make great strides.

Knowledge of neurological control of salivary secretion has formed the basis for novel therapeutic approaches. Salivary secretion is regulated by a reflex arch that consists of afferent receptors. Nerves carry impulses induced by actions on sialogogic gustation and mastication; a central connecting and processing salivation centre; and an efferent pathway consisting of parasympathetic and sympathetic autonomic nerve bundles that innervate the blood vessels and acini of their target glands [72]. It is believed that afferent nerves carry impulses to the salivary nuclei in the medulla oblongata, which in turn directs signals to the efferent part of the reflex arch leading to initiation of salivation [73]. This forms the basis of using pilocarpine and cevimeline in clinical practice by rheumatologists [46]. In SS, muscarinic, receptor-blocking autoantibodies may have potential pathogenic and diagnostic utility [74]. There is a suggestion that the sicca component of the SS may not be caused by irreversible structural damage of the secretory acinar cells but at least to some extent, by reversible functional perturbation which may be treatable [75].

Electrostimulation of neural and muscular structures is of therapeutic potential in several areas of medicine such as in pacemakers, phrenic stimulators, etc. A similar approach could potentially be applied to the management of salivary gland hypofunction. Theoretically, applying electrical impulses to components of the salivary reflex arch should result in improvement of salivary secretion. Animal studies have pointed towards the utility of this approach [76]. Schneyer and Hall showed that electric neurostimulation in the rat is a better approach as compared to pilocarpine for stimulating salivary secretion via reflex stimulation [77]. Also, stimulation of afferent neuronal receptors and pathways by application of an electrical current via the oral mucosa increased salivary production and lessened xerostomia in patients with salivary gland hypofunction [78]. Use of transcutaneous electric nerve stimulation (TENS) over the parotid gland has been reported to increase saliva production in healthy individuals and in patients with radiation-induced xerostomia, suggesting direct stimulation of the auriculotemporal nerve, which is the efferent pathway for the parotid gland [79]. Effects of electrostimulation were sustained for 6 months despite cessation of therapy in some patients, and this suggested that electrostimulation of nerves might release chemicals which promote regeneration of functional tissue [80]. This assumption is based on animal studies and in recent years advances have been made in the development of a new generation of intraoral devices, which, may revolutionize the management of xerostomia.

To exploit the principle of neuro-electrostimulation to increase salivary secretion, a first attempt led to the production of a device that was marketed in the USA (Salitron; Biosonics, Fort Washington, PA, USA). A probe was applied between the dorsum of the tongue and palate for a few minutes each day which delivered a stimulating signal to sensitive neurons of the mouth to induce salivation. This neuro-electrostimulation, when delivered repeatedly, led to an immediate response resulting in increased salivation and long-term response of sustained increase of salivary flow rate. This also resulted in a subjective improvement in xerostomia. The devise was approved by the US Food and Drug Administration in 1988 (PMA No. P860067). However, due to its large size, price and lack of user-friendliness, its widespread use was hampered. A second-generation salivary neuro-electrostimulator is GenNarino. This is a removable, horse-shoe shaped intraoral device embedded with electronic components and produced for individual patients for easy and safe self-use by using their teeth pattern molds and fits on the lower dentition. A remote control allows modification of its functions as per patient needs. The short-term effectiveness of the second-generation device was suggested in a randomized multicentre trial of patients with dry mouth from different causes [81]. The two outcomes of the study were measuring a decrease in oral dryness objectively by a built-in wetness sensor and subjective improvement of xerostomia-related symptoms. The device was well tolerated. There was significant moistening of the oral mucosal membranes as recorded objectively ($p < 0.0001$) and diminished xerostomia as reported subjectively ($p < 0.005$). This device was effective in reducing dryness of the mouth during application and up to 10 min after its removal [82]. Encouraged by this trial, a multinational study has been completed recently to assess the effectiveness of the device over a 12-month period [83]. The trial, entitled 'Safety and performance evaluation of an electro-stimulator mounted on an intra-oral removable appliance (GenNarino) for the treatment of xerostomia', was a prospective, randomized, double-blind, sham-controlled multi-centre trial, followed by an open-label study. This trial was designed to test the safety and efficacy of electrostimulation using the GenNarino device. The primary end-point is significant symptomatic improvement, and the secondary end-point is increased salivary output and event-free use. In stage I of the trial, the use of the device is compared in the active versus sham mode for 1 month each in a double-blind design. In stage II, the xerostomia-relieving effect of the active device is assessed in an open-label design for an additional 6 months. The results are awaited.

There may be a population of patients who may require more aggressive stimulation of the salivary glands, requiring trial of third-generation intra-oral devices. Saliwell Crown was developed, a permanently implanted oral cavity miniature neuro-electrostimulation device attached to a regular permanent dental implant located at the lower wisdom tooth area [71]. This device has an embedded wetness sensor. The crown can be renewed by a non-invasive technique at regular intervals. This crown is being tested in Europe [84]. The third-generation implantable device is able to deliver continuous or frequent stimuli, does not interfere with regular oral functions, has a wetness sensor to automatically change the intensity of stimulus and, at the same time, can be remote controlled. The implant is positioned in the region of the lower third molar to ensure close proximity to the lingual nerve that carries both afferent and efferent salivary impulses [78]. There are ongoing trials looking at the long-term effect of the third-generation neuro-electro-stimulator. If the results are promising, there may be a paradigm shift in the management of salivary hypofunction [85].

It is known that a significant level of apoptosis can be detected in the salivary gland cells after radiation treatment of the head and neck. This apoptosis has been suppressed in transgenic mice expressing an activated mutant of Akt (myr-Akt1) preclinical models. The serine/threonine protein kinase Akt, also known as protein kinase B (PKB). sup.1, provides an important survival signal in many different tissues [86]. Activation of Akt occurs in a PI3 kinase-dependent manner after stimulation of cells with a variety of growth factors that induce cell proliferation and cell survival. Potential substrates for Akt include procaspase, the pro-apoptotic Bcl-2 family member BAD and members of the Forkhead family of transcription factors [87]. Other recently identified substrates for Akt include tuberous sclerosis complex (Tsc2), a regulator of the mammalian target of rapamycin (mTOR), Myt1, a regulator of G2/M phase transition, YAP (Yes-associated protein), a transcriptional coactivator of the p53 homologue p73 and Chk1, a protein kinase activated by DNA damage whose activation is inhibited when phosphorylated by Akt [88]. It is well known that activated Akt suppresses apoptosis, although the *in vivo* mechanisms of this suppression are largely unknown. Akt can phosphorylate a number of substrates *in vitro*. However, the critical substrate(s) *in vivo* may depend on the cell type and stimulus [89]. In cases in which a clinical application of an inhibitor of apoptosis, according to the present invention, is contemplated, it will be necessary to prepare the complex as a pharmaceutical composition appropriate for the intended application. Generally, this will entail preparing a pharmaceutical composition that is essentially free of pyrogens, as well as any other impurities that could be harmful to living beings. Aqueous compositions of the present invention comprise an effective amount of the inhibitor of apoptosis, dissolved or dispersed in a pharmaceutically acceptable carrier or aqueous medium [90].

Such compositions are also referred to as inocula. The phrases 'pharmaceutically or pharmacologically acceptable' refer to molecular entities and compositions that do not produce an adverse, allergic or other untoward reaction when administered to an animal or human, as appropriate [91]. In the present context, 'pharmaceutically acceptable carrier' includes any and all solvents, dispersion media, coatings, antibacterial and antifungal agents, isotonic and absorption-delaying agents, and the like. The use of such media and agents for pharmaceutically active substances is well known in the field. Except insofar as any conventional media or agent is incompatible with the active ingredient, its use in the therapeutic compositions is contemplated. Supplementary active ingredients can also be incorporated into the compositions. Solutions of the active compounds as free base or pharmacologically acceptable salts can be prepared in water suitably mixed with a surfactant, such as hydroxypropylcellulose. Dispersions also can be prepared in glycerol, liquid polyethylene glycols and in oils. Under ordinary conditions of storage and use, these preparations contain a preservative to prevent the growth of microorganisms [92].

The inhibitor of apoptosis of the present invention may include classic pharmaceutical preparations. Administration of therapeutic compositions according to the present invention will be via any common route as long as the target tissue is available via that route. Administration could be by intradermal, subcutaneous, intramuscular, intraperitoneal, intra-arterial, or intravenous injections, intratumoral or regional to a tumour (salivary ducts, oral lavage) and systemic. Such compositions would normally be administered as pharmaceutically acceptable compositions that include physiologically acceptable carriers, buffers or other excipients [93].

Conclusion

Modern radiation techniques, salivary gland transfer and amifostine have shown promising results in preserving salivary gland function and have demonstrated a proven benefit in reducing both acute and chronic xerostomia. Amifostine is readily available in the clinic today, and IMRT technology is available increasingly in both academic and community radiation oncology practices. Salivary gland transplantation also appears to be promising, but further data are needed to ensure that this technique can be performed reliably in a multi-institutional setting. However, the advantage of one technique over the other is yet to be determined. Prospective trials need to be conducted to compare these modalities. A future key to preserving salivary function might involve a combination of all these measures. It is likely that several of the above therapies may be used to minimize damage to the salivary glands and maximize saliva after RT. Once these techniques become established, xerostomia may be less bothersome to these patients, who have already faced a very troublesome diagnosis.

References

1. Bjordal K, Kaasa S, Mastekaasa A. Quality of life in patients treated for head and neck cancer: A follow-up study 7 to 11 years after radiotherapy. *Int J Radiat Oncol Biol Phys* 1994;**28**:847–56.
2. Eisbruch A, Kim HM, Terrell JE, *et al.* Xerostomia and its predictors following parotid-sparing irradiation of head and neck cancer. *Int J Radiat Oncol Biol Phys* 2001;**50**:695–704.
3. Kaplan MD, Baum BJ. The functions of saliva. *Dysphagia* 2005;**8**:225–9.
4. Bahar G, Feinmesser R, Shpitzer T, *et al.* Salivary analysis in oral cancer patients: DNA and protein oxidation, reactive nitrogen species, and antioxidant profile. *Cancer* 2007;**109**:54–9.
5. Ship JA, Hu K. Radiotherapy-induced salivary dysfunction. *Semin Oncol* 2004;**31**:29–36.
6. Chao KSC, Low D, Perez CA, *et al.* Intensity-modulated radiation therapy in head and neck cancer: The mallincrodt experience. *Int J Cancer* 2000;**90**:92–103.
7. Parliament MB, Scrimger RA, Anderson SG, *et al.* Preservation of oral health-related quality of life and salivary flow rates after inverse-planned intensity-modulated radiotherapy (IMRT) for head-and-neck cancer. *Int J Radiat Oncol Biol Phys* 2004;**58**:663–73.
8. Eisbruch A, Ship JA, Martel MK, *et al.* Parotid gland sparing in patients undergoing bilateral head and neck irradiation: Techniques and early results. *Int J Radiat Oncol Biol Phys* 1996;**36**:469–80.
9. Kam MMK, Leung SF, Zee B, *et al.* Impact of intensity modulated radiotherapy (IMRT) on salivary gland function in early stage nasopharyngeal carcinoma patients: A prospective randomized study. *J Clin Oncol* 2007;**25**:4873–9.

10. Lee N, Xia P, Quivey JM, *et al.* Intensity modulated radiotherapy in the treatment of naso-pharyngeal carcinoma: An update of the UCSF experience. *Int J Radiat Oncol Biol Phys* 2002;**53**:12–22.

11. Tabak LA. In defense of the oral cavity: Structure, biosynthesis, and function of salivary mucins. *Annual Rev Physiol* 1995;**57**:547–64.

12. Liu R, Seikaly H, Jha N. Anatomic study of submandibular gland transfer in an attempt to prevent postradiation xerostomia. *J Otolaryngol* 2002;**31**:76–9.

13. Heck K. Prevention of radiation induced xerostomia and improved quality of life: subman-dibular salivary gland transfer. *Can J Med Radiat Technol* 2003;**34**:10–16.

14. Hodges D. Moving salivary glands may prevent dry-mouth. *Med Post* 2003;**39**:1–60.

15. Vineberg KA, Eisbruch A, Coselmon MM, *et al.* Is uniform target dose possible in IMRT plans in the head and neck? *Int J Radiat Oncol Biol Phys* 2002;**52**:1159–72.

16. Munter MW, Karger CP, Hoffner SG, *et al.* Evaluation of salivary gland function after treat-ment of head-and-neck tumors with intensity-modulated radiotherapy by quantitative pertech-netate scintigraphy. *Int J Radiat Oncol Biol Phys* 2004;**58**:175–84.

17. University of Washington Surgical Outcomes and Research. Copies of the UW-QOL Scale. Available at http://depts.washington.edu/soar/projects/dxcat/hnca/qol_uw.htm. Accessed March 1, 2005.

18. Bhatnagar A, Deutsch M. The role for intensity modulated radiation therapy (IMRT) in pedi-atric population. *Technol Cancer Res Treat* 2006;**5**:591–6.

19. Penagaricano JA, Papanikolaou N, Yan Y, *et al.* Application of intensity-modulated radiation therapy for pediatric malignancies. *Med Dosim* 2004;**29**:247–53.

20. Paulino AC, Skwarchuk M. Intensity-modulated radiation therapy in the treatment of children. *Med Dosim* 2002;**27**:115–20.

21. Teh BS, Mai WY, Grant WH 3rd, *et al.* Intensity modulated radiotherapy (IMRT) decreases treatment-related morbidity and potentially enhances tumor control. *Cancer Invest* 2002;**20**: 437–51.

22. Rembielak A, Woo TC. Intensity-modulated radiation therapy for the treatment of pediatric cancer patients. *Nat Clin Pract Oncol* 2005;**2**:211–17.

23. Huang E, Teh BS, Strother DR, *et al.* Intensity-modulated radiation therapy for pediatric medulloblastoma: Early report on the reduction of ototoxicity. *Int J Radiat Oncol Biol Phys* 2002;**52**:599–605.

24. Penagaricano JA, Yan Y, Corry P, *et al.* Retrospective evaluation of pediatric cranio-spinal axis irradiation plans with the Hi-ART tomotherapy system. *Technol Cancer Res Treat* 2007; **6**:355–60.

25. Jain N, Krull KR, Brouwers P, *et al.* Neuropsychological outcome following intensity-modulated radiation therapy for pediatric medulloblastoma. *Pediatr Blood Cancer* 2008;**51**:275–9.

26. Krasin MJ, Crawford BT, Zhu Y, *et al.* Intensity-modulated radiation therapy for children with intraocular retinoblastoma: Potential sparing of the bony orbit. *Clin Oncol (R Coll Radiol)* 2004;**16**:215–22.

27. Schroeder TM, Chintagumpala M, Okcu MF, *et al.* Intensity-modulated radiation therapy in childhood ependymoma. *Int J Radiat Oncol Biol Phys* 2008;**71**:987–93.

28. Jha N, Seikaly H, Harris J, *et al.* Prevention of radiation induced xerostomia by surgical trans-fer of submandibular salivary gland into the submental space. *Radiother Oncol* 2003;**66**:283–9.

29. Jha N, Seikaly H, Jacobs JR, *et al.* A phase II study of submandibular salivary gland transfer to the submental space prior to start of radiation treatment for prevention of radiation-induced xerostomia in head and neck cancer patients: RTOG 0244. Philadelphia: Radiation Therapy Oncology Group, American College of Radiology; 2003.

30. Seikaly H, Jha N, McGaw T, *et al.* Submandibular gland transfer: A new method of preventing radiation induced xerostomia. *Laryngoscope* 2001;**111**:347–52.

31. Suntharalingam M, Jaboin J, Taylor R, *et al.* The evaluation of amifostine for mucosal protec-tion in patients with advanced loco-regional squamous cell carcinomas of the head and neck (SCCHN) treated with concurrent weekly carboplatin, paclitaxel, and daily radiotherapy (RT). *Semin Oncol* 2004;**31**:2–7.

32. Brizel DM, Wasserman TH, Henke M, *et al.* Phase III randomized trial of amifostine as a radioprotector in head and neck cancer. *J Clin Oncol* 2000;**18**:3339–45.
33. Capizzi RL. The preclinical basis for broad-spectrum selective cytoprotection of normal tissues from cytotoxic therapies by amifostine. *Semin Oncol* 1999;**26**:3–21.
34. Korst AE, Sterre MLV, Gall HE, *et al.* Influence of amifostine on the pharmacokinetics of cisplatinum in cancer patients. *Clin Cancer Res* 1998;**4**:331–6.
35. Koukourakis MI, Kyrias G, Kakolyris S, *et al.* Subcutaneous administration of amifostine during fractionated radiotherapy: A randomized phase II study. *J Clin Oncol* 2000;**18**:2226–33.
36. Koukourakis MI. Subcutaneous injection of Ethyol: An alternative route of administration, in Abstract Book of a Satellite Symposium: Advances in Radiation Oncology. Presented at the 19th Annual Meeting of the European Society for Therapeutic Radiology and Oncology, Istanbul, Turkey, 2000 (abstr).
37. Hamlar DD, Schuller DE, Gahbauer RA, *et al.* Determination of the efficacy of topical oral pilocarpine for postirradiation xerostomia in patients with head and neck carcinoma [1994 annual meeting paper]. *Laryngoscope* 1996;**106**:972–6.
38. Johnson JT, Ferretti GA, Nethery WJ, *et al.* Oral pilocarpine for post-irradiation xerostomia in patients with head and neck cancer. *N Engl J Med* 1993;**329**:390–5.
39. Horiot JC, Lipinski F, Schraub S, *et al.* Post-radiation severe xerostomia relieved by pilocarpine: A prospective French cooperative study. *Radiother Oncol* 2000;**55**:233–9.
40. Warde P, O'Sullivan B, Aslandis J, *et al.* A phase III placebo-controlled trial of oral pilocarpine in patients undergoing radiotherapy for head and neck cancer. *Int J Radiat Oncol Biol Phys* 2002;**54**:9–13.
41. Zimmerman RP, Mark RJ, Tran LM, *et al.* Concomitant pilocarpine during head and neck irradiation is associated with decreased posttreatment xerostomia. *Int J Radiat Oncol Biol Phy* 1997;**37**:571–5.
42. Petrone, D, Condemi JJ, Fife R, *et al.* A double-blind, randomized, placebo-controlled study of cevimeline in Sjögren's syndrome patients with xerostomia and keratoconjunctivitis sicca. *Arthritis Rheum* 2002;**46**:748–54.
43. Guggenheimer J, Moore PA. Xerostomia: Etiology, recognition and treatment. *JADA* 2003;**134**:61–9.
44. Fife RS, Chase WF, Dore RK, *et al.* Cevimeline for the treatment of xerostomia in patients with Sjogren syndrome: A randomized trial. *Arch Intern Med* 2002;**162**:1293–300.
45. Nieuw Amerongen AV, Veerman EC. Current therapies for xerostomia and salivary gland hypofunction associated with cancer thera pies. *Support Care Cancer* 2003;**11**:226–31.
46. Porter SR, Scully C, Hegarty AM. An update of the etiology and management of xerostomia. *Oral Surg Oral Med Oral Pathol Oral Radiol Endod* 2004;**97**:28–46.
47. Markovic N, Abelson DC, Mandel ID. Sorbitol gum in xerostomics: The effect on dental plaque pH and salivary flow rates. *Gerodontology* 1998;**7**:71–5.
48. Rhodus NL, Brown J. The association of xerostomia and inadequate intake in older adults. *J Am Diet Assoc* 1990;**90**:1688–92.
49. Van Der Reijden WA, Vissink A, Veerman ECI, *et al.* Treatment of oral dryness related complaints (xerostomia) in Sjögren's syndrome. *Ann Rheum Dis* 1999;**58**:465–73.
50. Shahdad S, Taylor C, Barclay S, *et al.* A double-blind, crossover study of Biotène Oralbalance and BioXtra systems as salivary substitutes in patients with post-radiotherapy xerostomia. *Eur J Cancer Care (Engl)* 2005;**14**:319–26.
51. Sreebny LM, Schwartz SS. *A reference guide to drugs and dry mouth.* 2nd ed. *Gerodontology* 1997;**14**:33–47.
52. Pray WS. Consult your pharmacist. Help for patients with dry mouth. *US Pharmacist* 2000;**25**:16–22.
53. Epstein JB, Emerton S, Le ND, *et al.* A double-blind crossover trial of oral balance gel and biotene toothpaste versus placebo in patients with xerostomia following radiation therapy. *Oral Oncol* 1999;**35**:132–7.
54. Dirix P, Nuyts S, Vander Poorten V, *et al.* Efficacy of the BioXtra dry mouth care system in the treatment of radiotherapy-induced xerostomia. *Support Care Cancer* 2007;**15**:1429–36.

55. Dyke S. Clinical management and review of Sjögren's syndrome. *Int J Pharm Compound* 2000;**4**:338–41.
56. Ukai Y, Taniguchi N, Takeshita K, *et al.* Enhancement of salivary secretion by chronic anethole trithione treatment. *Arch Int Pharmacodyn Ther* 1988;**294**:248–58.
57. Hamada T, Nakane T, Kimura T, *et al.* Treatment of xerostomia with the bile secretion-stimulant drug anethole trithione: A clinical trial. *Am J Med Sci* 1999;**318**:146–51.
58. DRUGDEXÒ Editorial Staff. Yohimbine therapy of xerostomia (Drug Consult). In: Hutchison TA, Shahan DR, Anderson ML (eds). DRUGDEXÒ System. MICROMEDEX, Inc., Englewood (CO), edition expires 3/31/01.
59. Bagheri H, Schmitt L, Berlan M, *et al.* A comparative study of the effects of yohimbine and anetholtrithione on salivary secretion in depressed patients treated with psychotropic drugs. *Eur J Clin Pharmacol* 1997;**52**:339–42.
60. Aass N, DeMoulder PH, Mickisch GH *et al.* Randomized phase II/III trial of interferon alpha 2A with and without 13 cisretinoic acidin patients with renal cell cancer EORTC (30951). *J Clin Oncol* 2005;**23**:4172–8.
61. Yamada S, Mori K, Matsuo K, *et al.* Interferon alfa treatment for Sjogren's syndrome associated neuropathy. *J Neurol Neurosurg Psychiatry* 2005;**76**:576–8.
62. La Vecchia C. Mouthwash and oral cancer risk. *Oral Oncology* 2009;**45**:198–200.
63. Johnstone PAS, Riffenburgh RH, Niemtzow RC. Acupuncture for xerostomia: Clinical update. *Cancer* 2002;**94**:1151–6.
64. Blom M, Davidson I, Fernberg JO, *et al.* Acupuncture treatment of patients with radiation-induced xerostomia. *Eur J Cancer B Oral Oncol* 1996;**32B**:182–90.
65. Blom M, Lundeberg T. Long-term follow-up of patients treated with acupuncture for xerostomia and the influence of additional treatment. *Oral Dis* 2000;**6**:15–24.
66. Thomson WM, Williams SM. Further testing of the xerostomia inventory. *Oral Surg Oral Med Oral Pathol Oral Radiol Endod* 2000;**89**:46–50.
67. Thomson WM, Chalmers JM, Spencer AJ, *et al.* The Xerostomia Inventory: A multiitem approach to measuring dry mouth. *Community Dent Health* 1999;**16**:12–17.
68. Johnstone PAS, Peng YP, May BC, *et al.* Acupuncture for pilocarpine-resistant xerostomia following radiotherapy for head and neck malignancies. *Int J Radiat Oncol Biol Phys* 2001;**50**:353–7.
69. Cheng Xinnong. *Chinese acupuncture and moxibustion* (3rd ed. 2010). Foreign Language Press. China International Publishing Group, 24 Baiwanzhuang Str., Xicheng District, Beijing 100037, China.
70. Fargas-Babjak AM, Pomeranz B, Rooney PJ. Acupuncture-like stimulation with codetron for rehabilitation of patients with chronic pain syndrome and osteoarthritis. *Acupunct Electrother Res* 1992;**17**:95–105.
71. Wong RKW, Jones GE, Sagar SM, *et al.* A phase I-II study in the use of acupuncture like transcutaneous nerve stimulation in the treatment of radiation-induced xerostomia in head-and-neck cancer patients treated with radical radiotherapy. *Int J Radiat Oncol Biol Phys* 2003;**57**:472–80.
72. Proctor GB, Carpenter GH. Regulation of salivary gland function by autonomic nerves. *Auton Neurosci* 2007;**133**:3–18.
73. Murakami T, Ishizuka K, Uchiyama M. Convergence of excitatory inputs from the chorda tympani, glossopharyngeal and vagus nerves onto superior salivatory nucleus neurons in the cat Original Research Article. *Neuroscience Letters* 1989;**105**:96–100.
74. Fox RI, Konttinen Y, Fisher A. Use of muscarinic agonists in the treatment of Sjögren's syndrome. *Clin Immunol* 2001;**101**:249–63.
75. Jonsson R, Gordon TP, Konttinen YT. Recent advances in understanding molecular mechanisms in the pathogenesis and antibody profile of Sjögren's syndrome. *Curr Rheumatol Rep* 2003;**5**:311–16.
76. Izumi H, Karita K. Low-frequency subthreshold sympathetic stimulation augments maximal reflex parasympathetic salivary secretion in cats. *Am J Physiol* 1995;**268**:R1188–95.
77. Schneyer CA, Hall HD. Comparison of rat saliva's evoked by auriculo-temporal and pilocarpine stimulation. *Am J Physiol* 1965;**209**:484–8.

78. Steller M, Chou L, Daniels TE. Electrical stimulation of salivary flow on patients with Sjogren's syndrome. *J Dent Res* 1988;**67**:1334–7.
79. Schneyer CA, Humphreys-Beher MG, Hall HD, *et al.* Mitogenic activity of rat salivary glands after electrical stimulation of parasympathetic nerves. *Am J Physiol* 1993;**264**:G935–8.
80. Talal N, Quinn JH, Daniels TE. The clinical effects of electrostimulation on salivary function of Sjogren's syndrome patients. A placebo controlled study. *Rheumatol Int* 1992;**12**:43–5.
81. Clinical trial titled 'Evaluation of an Electro-Stimulator for the Treatment of Xerostomia (GenNarino)', ClinicalTrials.gov Identifier: NCT00509808. [Cited 2008 April 21].
82. Strietzel FP, Martín-Granizo R, Fedele S, *et al.* Electro-stimulating device in the management of xerostomia. *Oral Dis* 2007;**13**:206–13.
83. Saliwell Ltd, Wolff A. Evaluation of an electro-stimulator for the treatment of Xerostomia (GenNarino). ClinicalTrials.gov June 21, 2010. Identifier: NCT00509808.
84. Ami S, Wolff A. Implant-supported electrostimulating device to treat xerostomia: A preliminary study. *Clin Implant Dent Relat Res* 2010;**12**:62–71. Epub 2009 Aug 9.
85. Fedele S, Wolff A, Strietzel F, *et al.* Neuro-electro-stimulation in treatment of hypo salivation and Xerostomia in Sjögren. *J Rheumatol* 2008;**35**:1489–94.
86. Inoki K, Zhu T, Guan KL. TSC2 mediates cellular energy response to control cell growth and survival. *Cell* 2003;**115**:577–90.
87. Henry MK, Lynch JT, Eapen AK, *et al.* DNA damage-induced cell-cycle arrest of hematopoietic cells is overridden by activation of the PI-3 kinase/Akt signaling pathway. *Blood* 2001;**98**:834–41.
88. Humphries MJ, Limesand KH, Schneider JC, *et al.* Suppression of apoptosis in the protein Kinase C {delta} null mouse *in vivo. J Biol Chem* 2006;**281**:9728–37.
89. Burdelya LG, Krivokrysenko VI, Tallant TC, *et al.* An agonist of toll-like receptor 5 has radioprotective activity in mouse and primate models. *Science* 2008;**320**:226–30.
90. Garcia-Barros M, Paris F, Cordon-Cardo C, *et al.* Tumor response to radiotherapy regulated by endothelial cell apoptosis. *Science* 2003;**300**:1155–9.
91. Hiramatsu Y, Nagler RM, Fox PC, *et al.* Rat salivary gland blood flow and blood-to-tissue partition coefficients following X-irradiation. *Arch Oral Biol* 1994;**39**:77–80.
92. Sholley MM, Sodicoff M, Pratt NE. Early radiation injury in the rat parotid gland. Reaction of acinar cells in vascular endothelium. *Lab Invest* 1974;**31**:340–54.
93. Lin AL, Johnson DA, Wu Y, *et al.* Measuring short-term [gamma]-irradiation effects on mouse salivary gland function using a new saliva collection device. *Arch Oral Biol* 2001;**46**:1085–9.

Systemic Therapies in the Management of Head and Neck Cancer

Andrew W. Maksymiuk

Introduction

The management of head and neck cancer (HNC) is evolving with the introduction of more effective treatment strategies. Current optimal treatment strategies incorporate principles of best practices and practice guidelines [1]. Predictive factors, such as age, stage, co-morbidity and human papillomavirus (HPV) status have been shown to relate to outcome, thus making for a more accurate estimation of prognosis. Factor analysis has the validity to assess the potential for cure as well as palliative end-points, such as time to treatment failure and estimated survival [2–5].

Not all patients are suitable for 'aggressive' or 'radical' therapy, the successful application of which is limited to patients without significant co-morbidities, such as chronic obstructive pulmonary disease (COPD), liver disease from alcohol ingestion, heart disease, diabetes and advanced age. 'Aggressive' and 'radical' are terms that define curative intent, correlating with the potential for long-term survival. Radical combined-modality systemic therapy (chemotherapy)-radiotherapy (CRT) has been shown to result in an incremental improvement in outcome in patients with advanced-stage disease in the range of 5–8 % [6]. However, elderly patients and those with significant physiological impairments may suffer inordinately from toxicities [7–9]. Severe morbidity, even mortality, can result from overzealous application of aggressive, combined-modality treatment in marginal cases.

Many challenging questions remain or have been only partially addressed. For instance, the choice of systemic therapy for patients outside a clinical trial and its most effective and rational integration with radiation therapy for patients with advanced-stage disease is unresolved. Also, the age at which a patient is considered 'too elderly' for aggressive treatment has not been well defined. What constitutes physiological

A.W. Maksymiuk
Medical Oncology, CancerCare Manitoba, Department of Internal Medicine,
University of Manitoba, 675 McDermot Avenue, Winnipeg, MB, Canada
e-mail: andrew.maksymiuk@cancercare.mb.ca

© The Author(s) 2012
K.A. Pathak, R.W. Nason (eds.), *Controversies in Oral Cancer*,
Head and Neck Cancer Clinics, DOI 10.1007/978-81-322-2574-4_8

impairment significant enough to curtail aggressive combined-modality treatment, and how much compromise is acceptable in therapeutic strategy in a world of stringent treatment guidelines, remain unanswered. How best to minimize acute and chronic toxicities associated with aggressive therapy are important challenges.

Diagnostics

Positron emission tomography (PET) offers the potential for improved accuracy of staging patients with HNC and permits more accurate restaging after completion of combined modality therapy. For many anatomical sites, PET has succeeded in reducing the proportion of unsuccessful surgical interventions in patients with unsuspected metastatic disease. For HNC, this technology offers potential to refine our ability to select patients appropriately for aggressive therapy and ensure that all disease has been included in the treatment field or plan. Potentially, identification of residual disease could guide successful resection upon completion of CRT [10–13]. Additionally, PET has been found to be one of the strongest prognostic factors for disease-free survival and overall survival [10]. Patients with more extensive or metastatic disease can be identified and thereby unnecessary and toxic treatments that cannot achieve a curative outcome can be avoided.

In HNC, PET is currently associated with a higher rate of false-positivity in the regional lymph nodes because of the hypermetabolism associated with benign reactivity [10]. As reports are inconsistent, PET must be considered a promising emerging technology with a potential role, yet to be fully defined—particularly challenging for those patients with clinically node-negative disease.

Biological Markers and Molecular Indicators

Great interest has been shown in the potential of molecular markers, the signature of DNA mutations in HNC, which might be useful in prognosis or in selection of patients for specific therapies. For example, p16, p53, cyclin over-expression, ras and epidermal growth factor receptor (EGFR) mutations have been identified as promising molecular indicators for these purposes [14]. While it is tempting to include this information in devising a therapeutic plan, testing has not yet been standardized or become reliable enough for routine clinical use, beyond acting as stratification factors for clinical trials. Hopefully, some markers will be confirmed eventually as independent prognostic factors with important clinical relevance, but it is likely others will simply correlate with known clinical features.

Risk Factors

The relationship between co-morbidities, age, stage and location of cancer with outcome has been explored in retrospective analyses. These factors appear to be interactive to some degree. It has been suggested that the Charlson co-morbidity index should be included in all clinical research and therapeutic studies to prospectively clarify their role in outcome of treatment [8]. Meta-analysis of the role of systemic therapy indicates a diminution of the impact of systemic therapy with increasing age of the patients, with those >71 years of age apparently not achieving added benefit with this approach [6]. This effect could be explained by the increased toxicity experienced with chemotherapy in older age because of reduced metabolism and renal clearance of cytotoxics, poor tolerance of complicating infections, nutritional challenges and dehydration [15].

General recognition of HPV as an important emerging risk factor for the development of HNC has generated interest in determining if this virus is also a prognostic factor. It appears that patients with HPV-related tumours may have a better prognosis than patents whose tumours generated from 'conventional' carcinogens, such as cigarette smoke and alcohol [16]. For most new clinical trials, HPV is considered a stratification factor prior to assignment of the treatment arm. Whether or not treatment decisions should be different for patients with HPV-positive tumours is as yet undetermined. There are suggestions that targeted agents such as cetuximab may be more effective as systemic treatment in HPV-related tumours compared with tumours associated with other carcinogens [17]. Perhaps it will be possible to reduce the intensity of treatment in HPV-positive cases. Application of HPV vaccines to risk groups and/or as an immuno-adjuvant after treatment are tantalizing ideas.

Therapeutics

Systemic Therapy

Systemic therapy alone cannot be considered definitive for patients with HNC. Primary surgery may be very challenging or simply not feasible for treatment of patients with large primary tumours, extensive neck node metastases, extension to vital structures or significant co-morbidity. The concept of 'organ preservation' has become a feasible alternative in many patients who might have been treated surgically in the past. In these cases, the question of introducing chemotherapy as the initial therapy (induction therapy) is sometimes raised. This approach offers the potential to reduce the size of the primary tumour, thereby possibly improving the chances of success of RT for patients with advanced-stage disease.

Until recently, results of induction therapy trials have been disappointing [6]. Various regimens have been investigated, including familiar combinations of cisplatin plus 5-fluorouracil (5-FU). Combinations with the taxanes (paclitaxel, docetaxel) have been explored more recently [18–20]. Response rates are very high. In the past few years, results of induction chemotherapy trials with 3-drug regimens have been encouraging, with a reported improvement in time to treatment failure and, in some studies, survival [21–26]. Definition of the optimal induction regimen, identification of appropriate patient populations, and the role for concomitant CRT after induction therapy need clarification by confirmatory studies before establishing this approach as the standard.

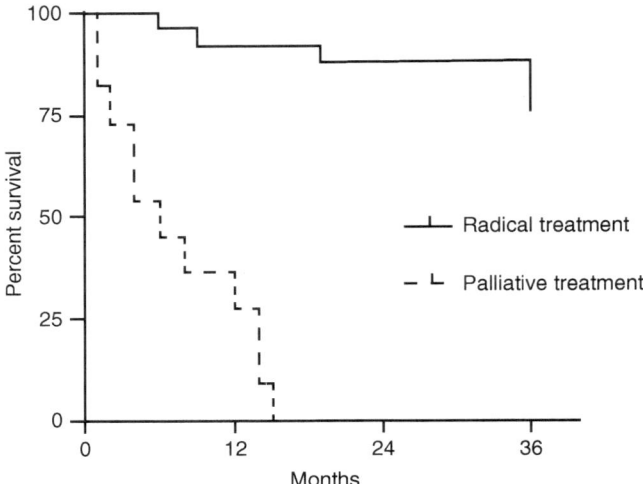

Fig. 8.1 Survival in advanced stage [III, IV] head and neck cancer. Data from 37 sequential patients treated with cisplatin, 5-FU+leucovorin 'induction' therapy with concomitant cisplatin+RT vs palliatively treated patients of similar stage (author's series)

Optimal Induction and Concomitant Treatment

The backbone of systemic therapy for HNC is cisplatin. Conventionally, the combination of cisplatin and 5-FU is considered standard induction therapy for HNCs, based on work from Wayne State University, USA, the Radiation Therapy Oncology Group (RTOG), and Dr M. Al-Sarraf and colleagues [27–30]. This approach has been moderately successful in improving the prognosis of patients with advanced-stage HNC. From meta-analysis, concomitant or alternating CRT was identified as having a better outcome defined by hazard ratio, compared with the neoadjuvant approach [6]. Responses and improvement rates are high with concomitant therapy, with cure rates in the range of 50–70 % reported in aggressively treated patients.

As an example, results from the author's selected clinical case series are depicted in Fig. 8.1 [unpublished data]. Patients were treated with two cycles of induction cisplatin+bolus 5-FU+leucovorin CT followed by cisplatin at 50 mg/m^2 every 2 weeks during the course of RT. In this series, the palliative group was defined when co-morbidities and tumour characteristics were unfavourable and RT doses were <4000 cGy.

Integration of taxanes and fluoropyrimidines with concurrent RT has been attempted with mixed results, mainly limited by excessive toxicity [31].

Pharmacokinetic and Dose-Schedule Considerations

Cisplatin has a proven track record for having an acceptable toxicity profile, in terms of locoregional toxicity, in conjunction with RT. Randomized controlled trials clearly demonstrate the improved efficacy of this combination therapy approach. The most common dose-schedule is 75–100 mg/m^2 at intervals of 3 weeks during RT; however, daily, weekly and every second-week schedules have also been employed with success. The rationale is that cisplatin is synergistic or additive to the effects of RT. Application of a high-dose schedule is associated with risks of significant systemic toxicity, such as nephropathy, neuropathy, diarrhoea and myelosuppression. *In vitro* studies suggest that a concentration of 1–2.5 μmolar of cisplatin in conjunction with RT is effective in achieving optimal cell-kill [32, 33]. Theoretically, the systemic agent should be available and circulating during the application of radiation to achieve the desired outcome. The relatively long half-life of cisplatin (5.4 days) would suggest that a lower dose given weekly or on a 2-weekly schedule could optimize the pharmacokinetic and toxicity characteristics of this agent [34]. Pharmacokinetic characteristics alone may be simplistic in terms of the biological effect of cytotoxic agents. In evaluating tissue levels of cisplatin, for example, residual tissue-level concentrations can be detected months after a single dose is administered. It has been postulated that the beneficial effects of concomitant cisplatin chemotherapy may be related more to the total dose of this agent administered during the course of RT than to the dose-schedule [6].

The other commonly used agent in the treatment of HNC is 5-FU. This agent has a short t$^{1/2}$ and for this reason, historically, has been administered on a daily ×5 bolus regimen. Several strategies have been evaluated to improve the therapeutic efficacy of 5-FU. Providing a constant blood level by continuous intravenous infusion (CIVI) is an approach that appears to improve efficacy and the effect of concurrent RT compared with bolus administration. In the treatment of colon cancer, infusions of 5-FU have been shown to be more efficacious than bolus schedules, although inconsistency exists [35, 36]. The apparent improvement in antitumour efficacy is associated with different or increased toxicities such as hand-foot syndrome, stomatitis, diarrhoea, dermatitis and coronary vasospasm, which are more common and myelosuppression, which is less common, with CIVI. Also, complications can occur with the requisite vascular access lines, ports and pumps, including increased infection risk and phlebitis/thrombosis with CIVI therapy [37]. Significant stomatitis is a side-effect of RT for HNC. The combination of 5-FU + RT may produce very severe and undesirable locoregional toxicities, whereas a combination of cisplatin with RT is better tolerated in terms of stomatitis.

Another important aspect of 5-FU is modulation of 5-FU cytotoxicity by other agents, such as leucovorin. The impact of leucovorin on the *in vivo* activity of 5-FU has been studied carefully [38]. Leucovorin modulates and increases cytotoxicity by enhancing thymidylate synthase inhibition, effectively shifting the metabolism of 5-FU from interaction with RNA towards the DNA pathway. The combination of 5-FU + leucovorin has been shown convincingly to be more efficacious than 5-FU alone [39]. However, this combination requires the dose of 5-FU to be reduced to avoid severe toxicity. Increased therapeutic efficacy is associated with increased toxicities, necessitating administration of a lower dose compared to single-agent 5-FU.

With most interventions, evidence from randomized controlled trials leads to changes in care standards. Randomized trials comparing 5-FU administered by

CIVI versus bolus schedules of 5-FU + leucovorin are difficult to find in the literature. With regard to HNC, existing studies indicate a benefit of bolus administration schedules. One study from South America indicated satisfactory palliative outcomes with a bolus regimen of cisplatin and 5-FU + leucovorin in advanced-recurrent squamous cell carcinoma (SCC) of the head and neck [40]. One European Organization for Research and Treatment of Cancer [EORTC] study compared two different schedules of 5-FU and RT for advanced-stage HNC. The bolus administration schedule coupled with RT resulted in a statistically insignificant improvement in outcome compared with the CIVI regimen [41]. In colon cancer, one published study from the Southwest Oncology Group (SWOG) demonstrated a non-significant benefit for bolus 5-FU + leucovorin versus CIVI [42]. In another, no benefit of 5-FU by CIVI + RT was demonstrable versus bolus 5-FU + RT. Toxicity was a major factor in discontinuing therapy with CIVI [37]. Nevertheless, most of the published studies on HNC are on the administration of 5-FU by CIVI, and this approach has become a standard of comparison in many randomized trials.

One method of minimizing toxicity is to reduce the dose of 5-FU. This strategy resulted in a more favourable toxicity spectrum for the 3-drug combination of docetaxel, 5-FU + cisplatin versus cisplatin + 5-FU in a recent study by Vermorken et al. [22]. Another recent phase II study by Fountzilas employed an induction regimen of docetaxel plus cisplatin without 5-FU with an excellent outcome [25]. If corroborated, the issue of the dose-schedule of 5-FU may become moot, questioning the need for 5-FU in any form as a component of induction treatment for HNC.

The addition of a taxane (either docetaxel or paclitaxel) increases the response rate compared with standard doublet therapy (Table 8.1). Improved time to treatment failure, locoregional control and survival have been reported recently with the 3-drug combination of taxotere (docetaxel), cisplatin + 5-FU (TPF) induction therapy leading to the conclusion that this 3-drug induction therapy should be the new 'standard' [23]. From these studies, it appears that the risk of severe side-effects, such as myelosuppression, nausea, mucositis and infection with 3-drug regimens can be moderated by attenuation of the dosage of 5-FU. Whereas not yet universally

Table 8.1 Induction regimens in head and neck cancer

Reference	Regimen	TTF/PFS (mos)	OS (mos)
Fountzilas et al. [18]	PacPF	11	16.7
Hitt et al. [24]	PF	12	37
	PacPF	20	43
Posner et al. [21]	PF	13	30
	TPF	36	71
Vermorken et al. [22]	PF	11.6	14.5
	RPF	15.4	18.8
Fountzilas et al. [25]	TP	16.4	24.4
Kies et al. [51]	Pac, Carbo + Cetux	>36	>36

PacPF paclitaxel, cisplatin + 5-fluorouracil, *PF* cisplatin + 5-fluorouracil, *TPF* docetaxel + cisplatin + 5-fluorouracil, *TP* docetaxel + cisplatin, *Cetux* cetuximab, *Carbo* carboplatin, *Pac* paclitaxel, *TPF* time to treatment failure, *PFS* progression-free survival, *OS* overall survival accepted, the strong renewed interest in induction therapy appears most likely to change the standard of care for a significant proportion of patients—particularly younger patients and those with good performance characteristics.

Consolidation Therapy

Similar to its role in nasopharyngeal cancer, 'consolidation' therapy may also be effective after definitive CRT in some patients with advanced-stage HNC. For most cancers, a minimum of four cycles of systemic chemotherapy is usually employed, with many regimens having 6 or even 8 cycles to achieve optimal benefit. A prerequisite for systemic chemotherapy to be efficacious is to use a regimen with at least a 30 % rate of inducing responses. If 'induction' + definitive CRT phases are considered to be analogous to a surgical intervention, then application of additional cycles of chemotherapy as 'consolidation' or 'adjuvant' therapy makes some sense in terms of potentially reducing the risk of relapse locally or at distant sites. Once patients have completed a course of radical concomitant CRT, they are often challenged nutritionally and in terms of locoregional toxicities, making application of additional cycles of chemotherapy problematic.

Systemic Therapy for Recurrent or Metastatic Disease

HNCs are known to be chemosensitive, although the duration of response to systemic therapy alone is usually short. Historically, many cytotoxic agents have been shown to have significant activity in advanced or recurrent HNC, including methotrexate, 5-FU, cis- and carboplatin, taxanes (paclitaxel and docetaxel), bleomycin and anthracyclines [19, 43, 44]. Combination chemotherapy may produce a higher response rate at the expense of increased toxicity but the impact in terms of survival benefit is less evident (Table 8.2). Although the combination of cisplatin + 5-FU is considered 'standard' in many centres, a randomized SWOG study indicated that methotrexate was equivalent to cisplatin + 5-FU [45]. More recently, the addition of 'targeted agents', such as

Table 8.2 Systemic therapy in head and neck cancer

Reference	Regimen	TTF/PFS (mos)	OS (mos)
Forastiere et al. [45]	Mtx	4	5.6
	P + 5-FU	4.2	5.0
	Carbo + 5-FU	5.1	5.6
Worden et al. [19]	PacP + 5-FU	4	10
Ferrari et al. [44]	Carbo + Pac	1	8
Vermorken et al. [54]	PI + 5-FU	3.3	7.4
	PI + 5-FU + Cetux	5.6	10.1

P cisplatin, *Carbo* carboplatin, *PI* cis or carboplatin, *5-FU* 5-fluorouracil, *Mtx* methotrexate, *Pac* paclitaxel, *Cetux* cetuximab, *TTF* time to treatment failure, *PFS* progression-free survival, *OS* overall survival

cetuximab, has resulted in improved response rates and survival compared with chemotherapy alone. The magnitude of benefit is of the order of a few months and,
although statistically significant, it is, however, of marginal clinical relevance. The
optimal dose, sequence and duration of treatment have yet to be defined.

New Drugs

HNCs have a high rate of expression of EGFR. Monoclonals, such as cetuximab,
panitumumab and other agents 'targeted' to block EGFR offer new avenues of therapy. Their favourable toxicity spectrum compared with conventional cytotoxic
agents makes them appealing for use in older patients and those with co-morbid
conditions that otherwise might make systemic therapy hazardous. These agents
have been administered in conjunction with RT and appear to produce outcomes
comparable to cytotoxic agents with less risk of significant systemic toxicity.
Cetuximab has also been administered in conjunction with conventional cytotoxic
agents in patients with recurrent or metastatic disease with encouraging results in
terms of response rates and survival [46–56]. 'Small-molecule'-targeted agents
(gefitinib and erlotinib) are also being investigated [57–60]. Responses within the
ranges reported for conventional cytotoxics have been reported with these agents in
small numbers of patients. Their role remains to be determined.

Selection of patients who could benefit most from application of targeted agents
versus less costly alternatives needs clarification. For example, encouraging results
have been reported with radiosensitizing agents, such as carboplatin in conjunction
with RT in small-scale trials [61]. Application of low-dose daily or weekly regimens
of cytotoxic therapy have also been advocated by some authors [62, 63]. The results
require confirmatory trials. These alternatives face challenges and perhaps are
unlikely to be validated because of the success and overwhelming interest in the
newer targeted therapies.

Systemic Therapy for the Carcinoma of Unknown Primary (CUP) Syndrome, Neck Presentation

This entity consists of two distinct subgroups: (1) SCC, which can have a good
prognosis and is usually treated similarly to SCC of other head and neck sites with
combined modality chemotherapy + RT, and (2) adenocarcinoma, a diverse group
[64, 65]. At autopsy and in later follow up, cancers of the thyroid, lung, gastrointestinal tract or other sites may be identifiable as primaries that have metastasized to
the neck. Studies, including immunohistochemistry, serum markers, PET scans and
aggressive therapy may yield positive results in a minority of cases. However, for
the majority, the prognosis is poor and the benefits of therapy are palliative rather
than curative. Recently, DNA micro-array technology and analyses of RNA have
been brought to bear in defining the primary site with encouraging preliminary
results [66]. Decisions are needed initially to direct a radical or potentially curative

strategy versus palliative management for patients presenting with CUP syndrome. Systemic therapy can be, and is often, a component of therapy in selected 'good performance' younger patients, although the benefit is difficult to predict or quantify through evidence-based trials or meta-analyses.

The application of complex and potentially toxic therapy may be justified if meaningful clinical benefit is likely, such as improved long-term survival or chance of cure. Exposing patients to the risk of significant toxicity is difficult to justify when the end-point is palliative and has a modest impact on survival. In such cases, conservative dose-schedules, attenuation of the duration of treatment and simplification of administration schedules can achieve the palliative objectives and avoid unpleasant side-effects and hospitalizations for toxicity.

Advanced Radiotherapy Techniques

Conventional 'fractionated field' radiotherapy is giving way to more sophisticated and specific modes of application, such as intensity-modulated radiation therapy (IMRT) and altered fractionation schedules, with hyperfractionation and/or concomitant boost techniques. These developments offer a higher dose application to the primary tumour and regional nodes while sparing local toxicities to normal regional structures. This reduces the toxicity risk for these patients [67–69]. Other new techniques, such as cyberknife or gamma-knife therapy may have improved efficacy compared to standard techniques. Safety and efficacy considerations with co-administration of systemic chemotherapy with these newer radiation techniques remain to be validated.

Supportive Care

Nutritional Support

Percutaneous endoscopic gastrostomy (PEG) tubes are often used to supplement oral diet in patients undergoing aggressive combined modality therapy for HNC. Some patients survive without PEG tubes; however, weight loss and fatigue can be alleviated and tissue healing promoted by adequate dietary support. A number of patients are able to tolerate aggressive therapy without the use of these tubes. Morbidity can be associated with placement of tubes, although techniques have improved. Some patients benefit by having PEG tubes available as a 'life-preserver' for use in the event of developing significant toxicities.

Xerostomia

A very common and significant long-term effect of radical therapy is loss or reduction in the function of the major and minor salivary glands, notably with RT, which damages them. This leads to disability in terms of mastication of food, swallowing, reduction in taste, and it also has implications in the preservation of dentition. Newer techniques of application of RT, such as IMRT, have reduced the severity of toxicity of RT by sparing some of the salivary glands from high doses of radiation. However, IMRT has not resolved the problem completely and many patients still face lifelong symptoms. Another approach is to surgically relocate one of the major salivary glands to outside the planned radiation field [70]. A multicentre randomized trial has demonstrated the efficacy of this intervention versus pilocarpine. As an additional surgical procedure is required, the impact of delaying initiation of RT and chemotherapy is unclear, but not likely to have much negative effect in an efficiently organized medical system.

Pilocarpine is a non-selective parasympathetic agent that promotes secretion of the salivary glands through stimulation of muscarinic receptors. This agent can be prescribed as therapy for xerostomia or during RT as a protective agent. It has demonstrated beneficial short-term effects in randomized trials. Frequent side-effects, such as sweating, headaches and increased urinary frequency, are disincentives. Also, caution is needed in patients with hypertension, COPD and in those taking concomitant medications. Because of its short duration of activity, pilocarpine requires regular administration for lengthy periods, which is cost-prohibitive for many patients. The overall impact on quality of life has been inconsistent in reported studies.

Amifostine is a radioprotectant agent developed to prevent toxicity from accidental radiation exposures. Its use has been advocated as a means to minimize subacute and chronic toxicities associated with therapeutic radiation. Acute stomatitis and chronic xerostomia remain significant morbidity considerations for HNC patients. Clinical studies have demonstrated an impact of amifostine on long-term xerostomia but rather surprisingly, not on the acute side-effects of radiation for head and neck cases [71, 72]. Cases of Stevens–Johnson syndrome have been reported with this agent and, although rare, this condition is unpredictable and can be life-threatening [73]. Furthermore, on the negative side, concerns have been expressed about the potential for protection of tumour cells from the therapeutic effects of radiation therapy by using amifostine. Its interactions with chemotherapy are unknown. Amifostine's cost is another consideration for restricting its routine use.

Anaemia

Combined modality treatment frequently has an impact on peripheral blood counts, producing anaemia, leukopenia, or thrombocytopenia. In most cases these effects are minor and require no specific intervention. Data suggest that RT may be less effective in anaemic patients. This is postulated to reflect diminished oxygenation of tumour cells, theoretically making them relatively hypoxic and thereby more resistant to cytotoxicity [74, 75]. In addition, anaemia has been found to be a negative predictor in terms of response in HNCs and other cancers. Transfusion of blood or packed cells is one way of alleviating this problem. Transfusion reactions such as fever, myalgias, allergic skin rashes and occasional transmission of viral or bacterial infections are inherent risks. For this reason, erythropoietin has been suggested as an alternative for maintaining a higher haemoglobin level. Erythropoietin, when administered to anaemic patients receiving chemotherapy, has been shown to improve symptoms such as fatigue. Haemoglobin levels and quality of life were shown to improve when erythropoietin was administered to patients with various cancers [76–78]. However, the impact of this approach on treatment outcomes is less clear.

The use of erythropoetin may increase the risk of pulmonary thrombo-embolism (sudden death) or possibly stimulate proliferation of malignant cells leading to reduced disease control time. Patient selection and trial designs make conclusive assessment problematic. Evidence of significant improvement in disease outcomes has been lacking in several studies investigating this approach.

New Directions

For the responsible utilization of new and improved technologies in diagnostics and therapeutics, a process is required to apply valuable resources to achieve maximal patient benefits. Linking databases to facilitate sharing of information between centres provides the potential for powerful realtime assessment and optimized patient outcomes. Multidisciplinary case conferences that combine the expertise of surgeons, radiation and medical oncologists, and other therapists provide an invaluable format to assess and decide on optimal therapeutic strategies for individual patients.

References

1. Pfister DG, Ang K, Brockstein B, *et al.* National Comprehensive Cancer Network. NCCN Practice Guidelines for Head and Neck Cancers. *Oncology (Williston Park)* 2000;**14**:163–94.
2. Argiris A, Karamouzls MV, Rabin D, *et al.* Head and *neck cancer. Lancet* 2008;**371**:1695–709.
3. Expanding role of the medical oncologist in the management of head and neck cancer. *CA: A Cancer Journal for Clinicians* 2008;**58**:32–53.
4. Marur S, Forastiere AA. Head and neck cancer: Changing epidemiology, diagnosis, and treatment. *Mayo Clin Proc* 2008;**83**:489–501.
5. Bhide SA, Nutting CM. Advances in chemotherapy for head and neck cancer. *Oral Oncol* 2010;**46**:436–8.
6. Pignon JP, le Maitre A, Maillard E, Bourhis J on behalf of the MACH-NC Collaborative Group. Meta-analysis of chemotherapy in head and neck cancer (MACH-NC): An update on 93 randomised trials and 17,346 patients. *Radiother Oncol* 2009;**92**:4(4–14).
7. Montoro JR, Hicz H, de Souza L, *et al.* Prognostic factors in squamous cell carcinoma of the oral cavity. *Rev Bras Otorrinolaringol* 2008;**74**:861–6.
8. Alho O-P, Hannula K, Luokkala A, *et al.* Differential prognostic impact of co-morbidity in head and neck cancer. *Head Neck* 2007;**29**:913–18.
9. Derksa W, de Leeuwb RJ, Jan Hordijka G. Elderly patients with head and neck cancer: The influence of comorbidity on choice of therapy, complication rate, and survival. *Curr Opin Otolaryngol Head Neck Surg* 2005;**13**:92–6.

10. Al-Ibraheem A, Buck A, Krause BJ, *et al.* Clinical applications of FDG PET and PET/CT in head and neck cancer. *J Oncol* 2009;208725.

11. Kyzas PA, Evangelos E, Denaxa-Kyza D, *et al.* 18F-Fluorodeoxyglucose positron emission tomography to evaluate cervical node metastases in patients with head and neck squamous cell carcinoma: A meta-analysis. *J Natl Cancer Inst* 2008;**100**:712–20.

12. Inokuchi H, Kodaira T, Tachibana H, *et al.* Clinical usefulness of [(18)] fluoro-2-deoxy-D-glucose uptake in 178 head-and-neck cancer patients with nodal metastasis treated with definitive chemoradiotherapy: Consideration of its prognostic value and ability to provide guidance for optimal selection of patients for planned neck dissection. *Int J Radiation Oncology Biol Phys* 2011;**97**:747–55.

13. Gourin CG, Boyce BJ, Williams HT, *et al.* Revisiting the role of positron-emission tomography/computed tomography in determining the need for planned neck dissection following chemoradiation for advanced head and neck cancer. *Laryngoscope* 2009;**119**:2150–5.

14. Egloff AM, Grandis JR. Improving response rates to EGFR-targeted therapies for head and neck squamous cell carcinoma: Candidate predictive biomarkers and combination treatment with Src inhibitors. *J Oncol* 2009;896407.

15. Ortholan C, Lusinchi A, Italiano AL, *et al.* Oral cavity squamous cell carcinoma in 260 patients aged 80 or more. *Radiother Oncol* 2009;**93**:516–23.

16. Goon PKC, Stanley MA, Ebmeyer AJ, *et al.* HPV and head and neck cancer: A descriptive update. *Head Neck Oncol* 2009;**1**:36.

17. Pajares B, Trigo Perez JM, Toledo MD, *et al.* Human papillomavirus (HPV)-related head and neck squamous cell carcinoma (HNSCC) and outcome after treatment with epidermal growth factor receptor inhibitors (EGFR inhib) plus radiotherapy (RT) versus conventional chemotherapy (CT) plus RT. *J Clin Oncol* 2011;**29** (suppl):367s, abstr 5528.

18. Fountzilas G, Tolis C, Kalogera-Fountzila A, *et al.* Paclitaxel, cisplatin, leucovorin, and continuous infusion fluorouracil for locally advanced squamous cell carcinoma of the head and neck. *Medical Oncol* 2005;**22**:269–79.

19. Worden FP, Moon J, Samlowski W, *et al.* A phase II evaluation of 3-hour infusion of paclitaxel, cisplatin, and 5-fluorouracil in patients with advanced or recurrent squamous cell carcinoma of the head and neck. *Cancer* 2006;**107**:319–27.

20. Colevas AD, Norris CM, Tishler RB, *et al.* Phase II trial of docetaxel, cisplatin, fluorouracil, and leucovorin as induction for squamous cell carcinoma of the head and neck. *J Clin Oncol* 1999;**17**:3503–11.

21. Posner MR, Hershock DM, Blajman CR, *et al.* Cisplatin and fluorouracil alone or with docetaxel in head and neck cancer. *N Engl J Med* 2007;**357**:1705–15.

22. Vermorken JB, Remenar E, van Herpen C, *et al.* Cisplatin, fluorouracil, and docetaxel in unresectable head and neck cancer. *N Engl J Med* 2007;**357**:1695–704.

23. Hitt R, Grau JJ, Lopez-Pousa A, *et al.* Final results of a randomized phase III trial comparing induction chemotherapy with cisplatin/5-FU or docetaxel/cisplatin/5-FU followed by chemoradiotherapy (CRT) versus CRT alone as first-line treatment of unresectable locally advanced head and neck cancer (LAHNC). *Proc Amer Soc Clin Oncol* 2009;**27 15S**:303s abst 6009.

24. Hitt R, Lopez-Pousa A, Martinez-Trufero J, *et al.* Phase III study comparing cisplatin plus fluorouracil to paclitaxel, cisplatin, and fluorouracil induction chemotherapy followed by chemoradiotherapy in locally advanced head and neck cancer. *J Clin Oncol* 2005;**23**:8636–45.

25. Fountzilas G, Bamias A, Kalogera-Fountzila A, *et al.* Induction chemotherapy with docetaxel and cisplatin followed by concomitant chemo-radiotheray in patients with inoperable non-nasopharyngeal carcinoma of the head and neck. *Anticancer Res* 2009;**29**:529–38.

26. Posner MR. Paradigm shift in the treatment of head and neck cancer: The role of neoadjuvant chemotherapy. *The Oncologist* 2005;**10**:11–19.

27. Jacobs JR, Pajak TF, Kinzie J, *et al.* Induction chemotherapy in advanced head and neck cancer. *Arch Otolaryngol Head Neck Surg* 1987;**113**:193–7.

28. Kish JA, Ensley JF, Jacobs JR, *et al.* Evaluation of high-dose cisplatin and 5-FU infusion as initial therapy in advanced head and neck cancer. *Am J Clin Oncol* 1988;**11**:553–7.

29. Department of Veterans Affairs Laryngeal Cancer Study Group. Induction chemotherapy plus radiation compared with surgery plus radiation in patients with advanced laryngeal cancer. *N Engl J Med* 1991;**324**:1685–90.

30. Al-Sarraf M, Martz K, Herskovick A, *et al.* Progress report of combined chemoradiotherapy versus radiotherapy alone in patients with esophageal cancer: An intergroup study. *J Clin Oncol* 1997;**1**:277–84.

31. Schrijvers D, Vermorken JB. Taxanes in the treatment of head and neck cancer. *Curr Opin Oncol* 2005;**17**:218–24.

32. Go RS, Adjei AA. Review of the comparative pharmacology and clinical activity of cisplatin and carboplatin. *J Clin Oncol* 1999;**17**:409–22.

33. Monk BJ, Burger RA, Parker R, *et al.* Development of an *in vitro* chemo-radiation response assay for cervical carcinoma. *Gynecol Oncol* 2002;**87**:193–9.

34. Havemann D, Wolf M, Gorg C, *et al.* Preclinical and clinical experience with cisplatin and carboplatin and simultaneous radiation in non-small cell lung cancer. *Ann Oncol* 1992;**3** [suppl3]:S33–S37.

35. De Gramont A, Bosset J-F, Milan C, *et al.* Randomized trial comparing monthly low-dose leucovorin and fluorouracil bolus with bi-monthly high-dose leucovorin and fluorouracil bolus plus continuous infusion for advanced colorectal cancer: A French intergroup study. *J Clin Oncol* 1997;**15**:808–15.

36. Budd GT, Flemming TR, Bukowski RM, *et al.* 5-fluorouracil and folinic acid in the treatment of metastatic colorectal cancer: A randomized comparison. A Southwest Oncology Group study. *J Clin Oncol* 1987;**5**:272–7.

37. Poplin EA, Benedetti JK, Estes NC, *et al.* Phase III Southwest Oncology Group 9415/Intergroup 0153 randomized trial of fluorouracil, leucovorin, and levamasole versus fluorouracil continuous infusion and levamisole for adjuvant treatment of stage III and high-risk stage II colon cancer. *J Clin Oncol* 2005;**23**:1918–25.

38. Grogan L, Sotos GA, Allegra CJ. Leucovorin modulation of fluororouracil. *Oncology (Williston Park)* 1993;**7**:63–72.

39. Meta-Analysis Group in Cancer. Modulation of fluorouracil by leucovorin in patients with advanced colorectal cancer: An updated meta-analysis. *J Clin Oncol* 2004;**22**:3766–75.

40. de Carvalho Fabricio V, Amado F, Del Giglio A. Low-cost outpatient chemotherapy regimen of cisplatin, 5-fluorouracil and leucovorin for advanced head and neck and esophageal carcinomas. *Sao Paulo Med J* 2008;**126**:63–6.

41. Lefebvre JL, Rolland M Tessellaar M, *et al.* Phase 3 randomized trial on larynx preservation comparing sequential vs. alternating chemotherapy and radiotherapy. *JNCI* 2009;**101**:142–52.

42. Leichman CG, Flemming TR, Muggia FM, *et al.* Phase II study of fluorouracil and its modulation in advanced colorectal cancer. A Southwest Oncology Group study. *J Clin Oncol* 1995;**13**:1303–11.

43. Volkes E, Stenson K, Rosen FR, *et al.* Weekly carboplatin and paclitaxel followed by concomitant paclitaxel, fluorouracil, and hydroxyurea chemotherapy: Curative and organ-preserving therapy for advanced head and neck cancer. *J Clin Oncol* 2003;**21**:320–6.

44. Ferrari D, Fiore J, Codeca C, *et al.* A phase II study of carboplatin and paclitaxel for recurrent or metastatic head and neck cancer. *Anti-Cancer Drugs* 2009;**20**:185–90.

45. Forastiere AA, Metch B, Schuller DE, *et al.* Randomized comparison of cisplatin plus fluorouracil and carboplatin plus fluorouracil versus methotrexate in advanced squamous cell carcinoma of the head and neck: A Southwest Oncology Group Study. *J Clin Oncol* 1992;**10**:1245–51.

46. Bonner JA, Harari PM, Giralt J, *et al.* Radiotherapy plus cetuximab for squamous-cell carcinoma of the head and neck. *N Engl J Med* 2006;**354**:567–78.

47. Caudell JJ, Sawrie SM, Spencer SA, *et al.* Locoregionally advanced head and neck cancer treated with primary radiotherapy: A comparison of the addition of cetuximab or chemotherapy and the impact of protocol treatment. *Int J Radiation Oncol Biol Phys* 2008;**713**:676–81.

48. Birnbaum A, Dipetrillo T, Rathore R, *et al.* Cetuximab, paclitaxel, carboplatin, and radiation for head and neck *cancer. Am J Clin Oncol* 2010;**33**:144–7.
49. Koukourakis MI, Tsoutsou PG, Karpouzis A, *et al.* Radiochemotherapy with cetuximab, cisplatin, and amifostine for locally advanced head and neck cancer: A feasibility study. *Int J Radiation Oncology Biol Phys* 2010;**77**:9–15.
50. Liu L, Cao Y, Tan A, *et al.* Cetuximab-based therapy versus non-cetuximab therapy for advanced cancer: A meta-analysis of 17 randomized controlled trials. *Cancer Chemother Pharmacol* 2010;**65**:849–61.
51. Kies MS, Holsinger FC, Lee JJ, *et al.* Induction chemotherapy and cetuximab for locally advanced squamous cell carcinoma of the head and neck: Results from a phase II prospective trial. *J Clin Oncol* 2009;**28**:8–14.
52. Buiret G, Combe C, Favrel V, *et al.* A retrospective, multicenter study of the tolerance of induction chemotherapy with docetaxel, cisplatin, and 5-fluorouracil followed by radiotherapy with concomitant cetuximab in 46 cases of squamous cell carcinoma of the head and neck. *Int J Radiation Oncol Biol Phys* 2010;**77**:430–7.
53. Bagust A, Greenhalgh J, Borland A, *et al.* Cetuximab for recurrent and/or metastatic squamous cell carcinoma of the head and neck: A NICE single technology appraisal. *Pharmacoeconomics* 2010;**28**:439–48.
54. Vermorken JB, Mesia R, Rivera F, *et al.* Platinum-based chemotherapy plus cetuximab in head and neck cancer. *N Engl J Med* 2008;**359**:1116–27.
55. Griffin S, Walker S, Sculpher M, *et al.* Cetuximab plus radiotherapy for the treatment of locally advanced squamous cell carcinoma of the head and neck. *Health Technol Assess* 2009;**13**:S49–S54.
56. Debucquoy A, Machiels J-P, McBride WH, *et al.* Integration of epidermal growth factor receptor inhibitors with preoperative chemoradiation. *Clin Cancer Res* 2010;**16**:2709–14.
57. Cohen EEW, Rosen F, Stadler WM, *et al.* Phase II trial of ZD1039 in recurrent or metastatic squamous cell carcinoma of the head and neck. *J Clin Oncol* 2003;**21**:1980–7.
58. Cohen EEW, Kane MA, List MA, *et al.* Phase II trial of gefitinib 250 mg daily in patients with recurrent and/or metastatic squamous cell carcinoma of the head and neck. *Clin Cancer Res* 2005;**11**:8419–24.
59. Kirby AM, A'Hern RP, D'Ambrosio C, *et al.* Gefitinib (ZD1839) as palliative treatment in recurrent or metastatic head and neck cancer. *B J Cancer* 2006;**94**:631–6.
60. Cohen EEW, Davis DW, Karrison TG, *et al.* Erlotinib and bevacizumab in patients with recurrent or metastatic squamous-cell carcinoma of the head and neck: A phase I/II study. *Lancet* 2009;**10**:247–57.
61. Homma A, Shirato H, Furuta Y, *et al.* Randomized phase II trial of concomitant chemoradiotherapy using weekly carboplatin or daily low-dose cisplatin for squamous cell carcinoma of the head and neck. *Cancer J* 2004;**10**:326–32.
62. Jeremic B, Shibamoto Y, Stanisavljevic B, *et al.* Radiation therapy alone or with concurrent low-dose daily either cisplatin or carboplatin in locally advanced unresectable squamous cell carcinoma of the head and neck: A prospective randomized trial. *Radiother Oncol* 1997;**43**:29–37.
63. Beckmann GK, Hoppe F, Pfreundner L, *et al.* Hyperfractionated accelerated radiotherapy in combination with weekly cisplatin for locally advanced head and neck cancer. *Head Neck* 2005;**27**:36–43.
64. Waltonen JD, Ozer E, Hall NC, *et al.* Metastatic carcinoma of the neck of unknown primary origin. Evolution and efficacy of the modern workup. *Arch Otolaryngol Head Neck Surg* 2009;**135**:1024–9.
65. Lenzi R, Hess KR, Aburzzese MC, *et al.* Poorly differentiated carcinoma and poorly differentiated adenocarcinoma of unknown origin: Favorable subsets of patients with unknown-primary carcinoma? *J Clin Oncol* 1997;**15**:2056–66.
66. Staub E, Buhr HJ, Grone J. Predicting the site of origin of tumours by a gene expression signature derived from normal tissues. *Oncogene* 2010 [Epub].

67. Tao Y, Daly-Schveitzer N, Lusinchi A, *et al.* Advances in radiotherapy of head and neck cancers. *Curr Opin Oncol* 2010;**22**:194–9.
68. Eisbruch A. IMRT reduces xerostomia and potentially improves QOL. *Nature Reviews Clin Oncol* 2009;**6**:567–8.
69. Milano MR, Vokes EE, Kao J, *et al.* Intensity-modulated radiation therapy in advanced head and neck patients treated with intensive chemoradiotherapy: Preliminary experience and future directions. *Intern J Oncol* 2009;**28**:1141–51.
70. Jensen SB, Pederson AML, Anderson E, *et al.* A systematic review of salivary gland hypofunction and xerostomia induced by cancer therapies: Management strategies and economic impact. *Support Care Cancer* 2010;**18**:1061–79.
71. Brizel DM, Wasserman TH, Henke M, *et al.* Phase III randomized trial of amifostine as a radioprotector in head and neck cancer. *J Clin Oncol* 2000;**18**:3339–45.
72. Koukourakis MI, Abatzoglou I, Sirridis L, *et al.* Individualization of the subcutaneous amifostine dose during hypofractionated/accelerated radiotherapy. *Anticancer Res* 2006;**26**:2437–43.
73. Valeyrie-Allanore L, Poulalhon N, Fagot J-P, *et al.* Stevens-Johnson syndrome and toxic epidermal necrolysis induced by amifostine during head and neck radiotherapy. *Radiotherapy Oncol* 2008;**87**:300–3.
74. Dische S. Radiotherapy and anaemia: The clinical experience. *Radiother Oncol* 2001;**20**:35–40.
75. Harrison LB, Chadha M, Hill RJ, *et al.* Impact of tumor hypoxia and anemia on radiation therapy outcomes. *Oncologist* 2002;**7**:592–608.
76. Glaspy J, Bukowski R, Steinberg D, *et al.* Impact of therapy with epoetin alfa on clinical outcomes in patients with nonmyeloid malignancies during cancer chemotherapy in community oncology practice. *J Clin Oncol* 1997;**15**:1218–34.
77. Witzig TE, Silberstein PT, Loprinzi CL, *et al.* Phase III randomized double-blind study of epoetin alfa compared with placebo in anemic patients receiving chemotherapy. *J Clin Oncol* 2005;**23**:2606–17.
78. Hoskin PJ, Robinson M, Slevin N, *et al.* Effect of epoetin alfa on survival and cancer treatment-related anemia and fatigue in patients receiving radical radiotherapy with curative intent for head and neck cancer. *J Clin Oncol* 2009;**27**:5751–6.

Surveillance After Treatment of Oral Cancer

Richard W. Nason and K. Alok Pathak

Introduction

Patients with cancer of the upper aero-digestive tract die from persistent or recurrent disease, second primary tumours, or intercurrent medical illness. In our experience with a cohort of 700 patients with oral cancer in the population-based tumour registry CancerCare Manitoba, 625 were treated with curative intent (R. Nason, 2010, unpublished data). Persistent disease was observed in 50 patients, the majority of whom were treated with radiotherapy (RT) as a single treatment modality. In the 575 patients that were rendered disease-free, recurrence was identified in 190 (30.4 %). The documented site of initial treatment failure was the primary site and neck in 117 and 82 patients, respectively. Distant metastases were observed at the time of initial treatment failure in 24 patients (3.8 %). Fifty-four patients (28 %) were rendered disease-free with further treatment. One hundred and fifty-seven second primary tumours were identified in 146 patients. The most frequent site was the head and neck ($n = 100$), followed by the lung ($n = 50$) and the oesophagus ($n = 7$). The overall and cause-specific survival at 5 years was 51 and 63 %. Overall survival by stage of disease was 74 %, 59 %, 52 % and 29 % for stages I–IV, respectively. The cause of death was documented in 336 of the 379 deaths observed in this cohort. Death was attributed to disease in 186 patients, new primary tumours in 70 and other causes in 80 patients [1]. These parameters are consistent with most reported series of oral cancer [2–6].

R.W. Nason
Department of Surgery, Faculty of Medicine, University of Manitoba,
ON2042 CancerCare MB 675 McDermot Avenue, Winnipeg, MB, Canada
e-mail: nasonrw@cc.umanitoba.ca

K.A. Pathak (✉)
CancerCare Manitoba, Department of Surgery, University of Manitoba,
Winnipeg, MB, Canada
e-mail: alok.pathak@cancercare.mb.ca

© The Author(s) 2012
K.A. Pathak, R.W. Nason (eds.), *Controversies in Oral Cancer*,
Head and Neck Cancer Clinics, DOI 10.1007/978-81-322-2574-4_9

Surveillance: Current Practice

Rigid and aggressive follow-up schedules have been prompted by the relatively high incidence of new tumour events, including both tumour recurrence and second primary tumours in patients with squamous cell carcinoma (SCC) of the upper digestive tract [1, 7, 8]. The assumption is that identifying and treating a new tumour event at an early and asymptomatic stage enables therapeutic options, improves survival and decreases cancer-specific morbidity [7, 8]. The frequency and duration of follow up varies between institutions and has not been standardized. In 1993, Marchant and coworkers reported the results of a survey of 290 members of the American Society for Head and Neck Surgery (ASHNS) [1]. Patients were followed on a monthly basis in the first year by 73 % of respondents. In the second postoperative year, patients were followed at a frequency of 2–3 months by 90 % of respondents. During postoperative years 3–5, patients were seen every 4–6 months by 97 % of respondents. All respondents reported seeing the patients either annually or semi-annually for the remainder of their lives. Eighty percent of respondents advocated the use of screening chest radiographs. The majority reserved head and neck imaging studies, such as CT scan and endoscopic examination under anaesthesia, for symptomatic patients.

In 1996, the ASHNS and the Society of Head and Neck Surgery (SHNS) collaborated to form a clinical guidelines task force resulting in a booklet of consensus guidelines (ASHNS, SHNS 1996). Surveillance guidelines are provided for the major tumour sites in the head and neck. These guidelines are now published as part of the NCCN (National Comprehensive Cancer Network) Clinical Practice Guidelines in Oncology [10] and have been endorsed by the American Head and Neck Society. They form the basis of follow up for the Head and Neck Disease Site Group at CancerCare Manitoba (Table 9.1). Each follow-up visit includes a needs assessment by nursing staff, completion of a quality-of-life survey, and clinical evaluation of the upper aero-digestive tract including fibre-optic nasal endoscopy as indicated. Assessment and intervention of speech language pathology, nutrition services, physiotherapy, and psychosocial oncology are directed by the needs assessment. Imaging studies (CT and/or MRI) are performed 6 weeks post-treatment and again in 6–12 weeks to establish stability of post-treatment changes. Following this patients are imaged as clinically indicated. In irradiated patients thyroid function is followed clinically with a TSH level performed annually.

Table 9.1 Follow-up visits per year post-treatment for patients with oral cancer at CancerCare Manitoba, Canada

	Years after treatment					
	1	2	3	4	5	5+
Number of visits[a]	6–8	4–6	3–4	3–4	3–4	1–2

[a]Visit includes needs assessment performed by nursing staff; completion of quality of life survey; evaluation of upper aero-digestive tract by physician with fibre-optic nasendoscopy as indicated; evaluation and intervention of speech language pathology, nutrition, physiotherapy, psychosocial oncology, as per needs assessment

Surveillance: Evidence For and Against

Evaluation of the efficacy of surveillance after treatment of head and neck cancer (HNC) is limited to several general and site-specific descriptive studies [1, 8, 9, 11–17]. Only one study was identified that was specific to the oral cavity [8]. The assumption challenged in these studies is that rigid, scheduled follow up can reduce cancer-related morbidity from new tumour events. In summary, the use of routine and rigid follow-up schedules in this patient population to reduce cancer-related morbidity is of limited benefit [1, 8, 9, 11, 15, 16]. The majority of recurrences are symptomatic and a significant proportion of patients with recurrence present on a self-referred basis. Two studies showed no difference in survival between patients presenting with symptoms and asymptomatic patients identified at the time of routine visits [8, 15]. In contrast, De Visscher and Manni reported improved survival and asymptomatic recurrences identified at the time of a scheduled visit [12]. It is noted, however, that these authors measured survival time from the time of treatment of the recurrence and not the time of treatment of the index tumour. This, therefore, confounded the results with lead-time bias [15]. It is estimated that only 2–3 % of asymptomatic recurrences benefit from routine follow-up visits [9, 15]. The limited treatment success observed was restricted to patients with early-stage disease treated with a single modality. This subset of patients tended to be amenable to further treatment options. In patients with advanced-stage disease, the probability of survival after a recurrence is negligible because no treatment options are available [6, 9, 13, 15, 16]. The majority of investigators questioned the necessity of follow up after 3 years and particularly beyond 5 years.

The use of chest X-rays on a routine basis during follow up has been questioned recently [18–20]. Ritoe et al. performed 2008 routine chest radiographs in high-risk HNC patients [18]. This was productive in 11 patients in whom a curative resection could be offered. Three of these patients derived a significant survival benefit. Additional studies have shown no benefit from routine chest radiographs [14, 15].

The role of routine surveillance in patients with SCC of the upper aero-digestive tract at CancerCare Manitoba has not been evaluated systematically. It is our clinical impression that the majority of recurrences in our practice are symptomatic. The poor survival of patients with recurrent disease is consistent with our own experience.

Conclusion and Future Directions

The objectives of surveillance and follow up after treatment of SCC of the upper aero-digestive tract extend beyond the objective of decreasing morbidity from new cancer recurrences. Requirements for rehabilitation are a major component of follow-up visits. These needs, in fact, will preclude a randomized trial to evaluate the efficacy of surveillance. Follow-up visits cannot be denied to any subset of patients. Surveillance is also important to document outcomes, which should be the evidence base for our therapeutic decisions [1].

Surveillance of HNCs post-treatment should continue by using the guidelines that have been presented. We do, however, feel that the goals of follow up need to be identified clearly, and that the emphasis of certain tasks should possibly be shifted away from physicians. In the majority of patients the intent of follow up should be care and not cure [1, 9, 15]. All patients require monitoring for complications of treatment, such as hypothyroidism resulting from irradiation of the neck. Most patients will require the help of speech language pathologists, nutritionists, physiotherapists and dental specialists. The psychosocial consequences of treatment of HNC are well recognized. In patients with early-stage disease who are treated with a single modality, surveillance is appropriate to identify recurrences that are potentially treatable. In patients with advanced-stage disease, the emphasis needs to be on managing and minimizing the consequences of recurrent disease when they occur. Surveillance of patients beyond 2–3 years is necessary to document treatment outcomes accurately. The emphasis of follow up should shift from a physician-based event to a multidisciplinary exercise that addresses the needs and expectations of the patient [1].

It is the authors' opinion that recurrent disease often indicates aggressive disease. Even an earlier diagnosis cannot guarantee that the ultimate outcome will not change. It needs to be emphasized that the studies presented are based on identification of recurrence on physical findings. Evidence shows that physical examination is inferior to imaging in certain aspects [21]. The sensitivity of physical examination in identifying cervical lymph nodes is ~50–60 %. Imaging studies, including MR, CT and ultrasound, are superior and able to identify 75–80 % of metastatic disease in the neck [21]. Nieuwenhuis and co-workers evaluated the use of ultrasound-guided cytological assessment of sentinel nodes in the management of the N0 neck [22]. Ultrasound was used as part of the follow-up assessment. During the follow-up period, 34/161 (21 %) developed lymph node metastases. These authors reported a salvage rate of 79 %, which is two to three times higher than that observed in our own experience. This suggests that Nieuwenhuis and co-workers were able to identify cervical node metastases that were more amenable to salvage treatment at an earlier stage. There have been qualitative assessments of the use of positron emission tomography (PET) in the follow up of patients with advanced HNC [23, 24]. Preliminary evidence suggests that PET may be useful in identifying residual or recurrent HNC. In our opinion, imaging needs to be introduced in a formal fashion into follow-up protocols. This aspect of surveillance would be amenable to a systematic assessment.

The outcome of patients with SCC of the upper aero-digestive tract is predominantly determined by the biology of the tumour. Treatment can modify the course of the illness. The ability to predict treatment outcome on the basis of the biology of the tumour would facilitate planning for surveillance. At present, the ability to stratify patients into high- and low-risk groups on the basis of clinical imaging and histopathological parameters does not permit refinement of the follow-up schedules [17]. Cancer is a consequence of genetic and epigenetic alterations at the cellular level. The use of molecular techniques to describe tumour-specific characteristics to predict the tumour phenotype would be of obvious benefit. This science is in its infancy. The study of DNA microarrays and genomic hybridization show promise.

Presently, however, no single marker, technique, or group of parameters is available which are sufficiently reproducible and sensitive for clinical use [25]. Structured surveillance programmes will, however, be necessary to evaluate the benefit of new prognostic indices [1].

References

1. Nason RW, Butler J. Upper aerodigestive tract carcinoma. A Canadian perspective. In: Johnson FE, Virgo KS, Margenthaler JA, *et al.* (eds). *Patient surveillance after cancer treatment: An international perspective.* Accepted for publication 2011.
2. Taneja C, Allen H, Koness RJ, *et al.* Changing patterns in failure of head and neck cancer. *Arch Otolaryngol Head Neck Surg* 2002;**128**:324–27.
3. Carvalho AL, Magrin J, Kowalski LP. Sites of recurrence in oral and oropharyngeal cancers according to the treatment approach. *Oral Diseases* 2003;**9**:112–18.
4. Vikram B. Changing patterns of failure in advanced head and neck cancer. *Arch Otolaryngol Head Neck Surg* 1984;**110**:564–5.
5. Dhooge IJ, De Vos M, Van Cauwenberge PB. Multiple primary malignant tumors in patients with head and neck cancer: Results of a prospective study and future perspectives. *The Laryngoscope* 1998;**108**:250–56.
6. Lippman SM, Hong WK. Second malignant tumors in head and neck squamous cell carcinoma: The overshadowing threat for patients with early-stage disease. *Int J Radiat Oncol Biol Phys* 1989;**17**:691–4.
7. Marchant FE, Lowry LD, Moffitt JJ, *et al.* Current national trends in the posttreatment follow-up of patients with squamous cell carcinoma of the head and neck. *Am J of Otolaryngol* 1993;**14**:88–93.
8. Matthias AW, van Gulick JJ, Marres HA, *et al.* Effectiveness of routine follow-up of patients treated for T1–2 N0 oral squamous cell carcinomas of the floor of mouth and tongue. *Head Neck* 2006;**28**:1–7.
9. Cooney TR, Poulsen MG. Is routine follow-up useful after combined-modality therapy for advanced head and neck cancer? *Arch Otolaryngol Head Neck Surg* 1999;**125**:379–82.
10. NCCN Clinical Practice Guidelines in Oncology 2008. http://www.nccn.org.
11. Haas I, Hauser U, Ganzer U. The dilemma of follow-up in head and neck cancer patients. *Eur Arch Otorhinolaryngol* 2001;**258**:177–83.
12. De Visscher AV, Manni JJ. Routine long-term follow-up in patients treated with curative intent for squamous cell carcinoma of the larynx, pharynx, and oral cavity. Does it make sense? *Arch Otolaryngol Head Neck Surg* 1994;**120**:934–9.
13. Boysen M, Lovdal O, Tausjo J, *et al.* The value of follow-up in patients treated for squamous cell carcinoma of the head and neck. *Eur J Cancer* 1992;**28**:426–30.
14. Grau JJ, Cuchi A, Trasserra J, *et al.* Follow-up study in head and neck cancer: Cure rate according to tumor location and stage. *Oncology* 1997;**54**:38–42.
15. Ritoe SC, Krabbe PF, Kaanders JH, *et al.* Value of routine follow-up for patients cured of laryngeal carcinoma. *Cancer* 2004;**101**:1382–9.
16. Ritoe SC, Bergman H, Krabbe PFM, *et al.* Cancer recurrence after total laryngectomy: Treatment options, survival, and complications. *Head Neck* 2006;**28**:383–8.
17. Ritoe SC, Verbeek ALM, Krabbe PFM, *et al.* Screening for local and regional cancer recurrence in patients curatively treated for laryngeal cancer: Definition of a high-risk group and estimation of the lead time. *Head Neck* 2007;**29**:431–8.
18. Ritoe SC, Krabbe PF, Jansen MM, *et al.* Screening for second primary lung cancer after treatment of laryngeal cancer. *Laryngoscope* 2002;**112**:2002–8.
19. Matthias AW, Boustahji AH, Kaanders JH, *et al.* A half-yearly chest radiograph for early detection of lung cancer following oral cancer. *Int J Oral Maxillofac Surg* 2002;**31**:378–82.

20. Shah SI, Applebaum EL. Lung cancer after head and neck cancer: Role of chest radiography. *Laryngoscope* 2000;**110**:2033–6.
21. Van den Brekel MW, Castelijns JA, Snow GB. Diagnostic evaluation of the neck. *Otolaryngol Clin North Am* 1998;**31**:601–20.
22. Nieuwenhuis EJ, Castelijns JA, Pijpers R, *et al.* Wait-and-see policy for the N0 neck in early-stage oral and oropharyngeal squamous cell carcinoma using ultrasonography-guided cytology: Is there a role for identification of the sentinel node? *Head Neck* 2002:**24**:282–9.
23. Goerres GW, Schmid DT, Bandhauer F, *et al.* Positron emission tomography in the early follow-up of advanced head and neck cancer. *Arch Otolaryngol Head Neck Surg* 2004;**130**:105–9.
24. Isles MG, McConkey C, Mehanna HM. A systematic review and meta-analysis of the role of positron emission tomography in the follow-up of head and neck squamous cell carcinoma following radiotherapy or chemotherapy. *Clin Otolaryngol* 2008;**33**:210–22.
25. Cheng AC, Schmidt BL. Management of the N0 neck in oral squamous cell carcinoma. *Oral Maxillofacial Surg Clin N Am* 2008;**40**:477–97.

Index

A
American Head and Neck Society 54, 116
American Society for Head and Neck Surgery
    (ASHNS) 116
American Society of Clinical Oncology 85

B
Bony defects, reconstruction of 66–7
Brazilian Head and Neck Cancer
    Study Group 54

C
CancerCare Manitoba 115,116t, 117
Charlson co-morbidity index 100
Clinical Practice Guidelines in Oncology 116.
    See also NCCN

E
Eastern Cooperative Oncology Group (ECOG)
    Trial 8
Elective neck dissection 53–5
    evidence in support of 53
Erythroplakia 26–7
European Organization for Research and
    Treatment of Cancer (EURTOC)
    Study 104
EXTREME (Erbitux in First-line Treatment
    of Recurrent or Metaststic Head
    and Neck Cancer) Trial 6

F
Food and Drug Administration (FDA) 5, 91
Free flaps 64–5
    anterolateral flap 65
    radial forearm flap 64, 64f

H
Hard palate defects 68. *See also* Oral reconstruction
Head and neck cancer (HNC)
    induction regimens 104,104t
    supportive care 107
        anaemia 108
        new directions 109
        nutritional support 107
        xerostomia 107
    systemic therapies 99–109, 105t
        biological markers and molecular
            indicators 100
        diagnostics 100
        risk factors 100
        therapeutics 101
    therapeutics
        consolidation therapy 105
        new drugs 106
        optimal induction and concomitant
            treatment 102
        pharmacokinetics and dose schedule 102
        systemic therapy 101
        systemic therapy for recurrent or
            metastatic disease 105
        systemic therapy for the carcinoma of
            unknown primary (CUP) syndrome,
            neck presentation 106
Head and Neck Disease Site Group,
    CancerCare (Manitoba) 116
Head and neck squamous cell carcinoma
    (HNSCC)
    molecular signatures 2
    molecular-targeted therapies 2–7
    molecular targets and their inhibitors for
        therapy 4–5
    non-surgical management 1
    personalized medicine 11
    prognosis 1
    targeted therapies 2

© The Author(s) 2012
K.A. Pathak, R.W. Nason (eds.), *Controversies in Oral Cancer*,
Head and Neck Cancer Clinics, DOI 10.1007/978-81-322-2574-4

Hepatitis C virus (HCV) infection 23
Human papillomavirus (HPV) 2, 18, 22, 25,
    99, 101
Human papillomavirus vaccines 9, 101

L
Leukoplakia 17–21
    cryo surgery 20
    definition of 17
    impact of HPV 18
    medical management 19, 21
    molecular diagnostic techniques 18
    photodynamic therapy 21
    prevalence of 18
    risk factors for 18
    surgical management 20
Locoregional flaps 63
    infrahyoid myocutaneous flap 63
    nasolabial flaps 63
    pectoralis major myocutaneous flap 63, 64t

M
Mandible
    reconstruction of 72
    sites of invasion 34f
    lip-split approach 36, 48
    lip-split mandibulectomy approach 36–8
    marginal mandibulectomy 38–42
    pull-through approach 38
    per-oral approach 36
    preserving alternatives 33–42
    preserving approaches to oral cancer 35–36
    transoral–transcervical approach 36–8
Mandibular defects, palate flap option 73t
Molecular targets for therapy of HNC 2–7
    biological-targeted agents for HNSCC 9
    from bench to bedside 1–11
    future strategies 10
    kinases (serine/threonine and tyrosine) 8–9
    PI3-K/Akt pathway 7–8
    and their inhibitors used for HNSCC
        therapy 4–5t
Mucosal defects, reconstructive options 62–5

N
NO neck in oral cancer, management of 51–8
National Comprehensive Cancer Network
    (NCCN) guidelines 116
Neck dissection. See Elective neck dissection

O
Occult metastases
    biological significance of 52
    predicting 52–3
Okay classification for reconstruction of
        palato-maxillary defects 69, 70t
Oral cancer
    factors determining the surgical
        approach 35t
    radiation for 79
    surgical management 45–8
Oral cavity
    potentially malignant disorders of 17–28
    reconstruction of, current options and
        controversies 61–74
Oral lichen planus 21–26
    drug-induced 22–4
    pathogenic link with HCV 23
    psychological profile of the patient 22
    treatment for 26–6
Oral reconstruction, controversies in 67–74
Oral submucous fibrosis 27–8

P
Palato-maxillary defects 69, 70t
Pectoralis major myocutaneous flap 68, 71, 72
Pedicled flap versus free flaps 71. See also Oral
        reconstruction
Primary closure/healing by secondary
        intention 62

R
Radial forearm flap 71
Radiation techniques, conformal 80–3
Radiation Therapy Oncology Group 82,
        84,102
Radiotherapy techniques, advanced 107
Reconstructive surgery, principles of 6, 62t

S
Salivary gland transfer, surgery 83
Salivary glands, preserving the function 79–93
    future considerations 87
    pharmacological considerations 84
    symptomatic approaches 87
Sensate flap 68. See also Oral reconstruction
Sentinel lymph node biopsy 55–8
Signalling pathways, deregulation of 2, 3f
Skin grafting 62

Society of Head and Neck Surgery (SHNS)
116
Southwest Oncology Group (SWOG)
104, 105
Submucous fibrosis. *See* Oral submucous
fibrosis
Surgical management, principles
of 47–8
Surgical resection margin 46–7
Surveillance after treatment of oral cancer
115–19
current practice 116
evidence for and against 117

T
Transoral laser microsurgery 62

W
WHO Collaborating Centre for Oral Pathology
and Precancer 17

X
Xerostomia 80–89
radiation-induced 80
use of acupuncture 89, 90